WHAT IS LIFE?

The path to an abundant, prosperous and happy life.

K.K.BHAMRA

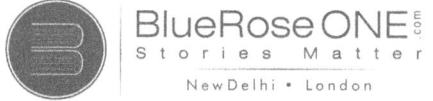

BLUEROSE PUBLISHERS
India | U.K.

Copyright © K. K Bhamra 2025

All rights reserved by author. No part of this publication may be reproduced, stored in a retrieval system or transmitted in any form or by any means, electronic, mechanical, photocopying, recording or otherwise, without the prior permission of the author. Although every precaution has been taken to verify the accuracy of the information contained herein, the publisher assumes no responsibility for any errors or omissions. No liability is assumed for damages that may result from the use of information contained within.

BlueRose Publishers takes no responsibility for any damages, losses, or liabilities that may arise from the use or misuse of the information, products, or services provided in this publication.

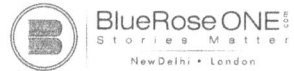

For permissions requests or inquiries regarding this publication, please contact:

BLUEROSE PUBLISHERS
www.BlueRoseONE.com
info@bluerosepublishers.com
+91 8882 898 898
+4407342408967

ISBN: 978-93-5989-534-5

Cover design: Shubham Verma
Typesetting: Sagar

First Edition: May 2025

Disclaimer

The content of this book is the personal experiences, learnings, and teachings of the author, which she has learned in her journey of life and are shared only with the intention to make the reader aware of how powerful and miraculous as a human we are, to be a creator of their own lives, and how they could reach their dreams and goals.

The images used in this book are derived from www.freepik.com, www.pexels.com, www.pixabay.com and www.unsplash.com. These websites have free copyright images. There is no intention of the author or the publishers to use copyrighted images. All images that are used in the book are purely with the intention that these are copyright-free and are used for the better understanding of the reader.

The quotes and references mentioned are sourced from Google, and the author and publishers do not own any liability in case it turns out to be incorrect. These quotes and references are used only with the intention of making content more authenticated, more reliable and more understandable to the reader.

The image of Water Experiment is an illustration and has not violated any copyrights.

To my higher self /My dear Subconscious mind/
The Divine powers of this Universe

With you giving me the strong impulse to start writing, I now, at this moment, hold my pen and journal to pen down what you want me to write to add value to the lives of others. I request that you guide me in my journey of writing this book, offering you my loving subconscious mind and calling out all the divine powers in this whole universe to guide me in writing this book, which could help in transforming the lives of millions who would read it with the intention to learn and transform their lives in the most positive way.

Thank you, Thank you, Thank you.

MY ACHIEVEMENTS

I feel more than blessed to share my achievements.

Apart from being a Master's of Laws (LLM) I succeeded in becoming **"Forever Star Mrs Amritsar 2024"** (City Winner).

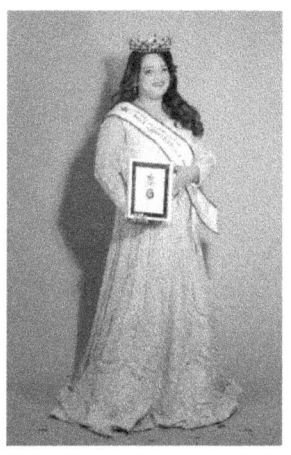

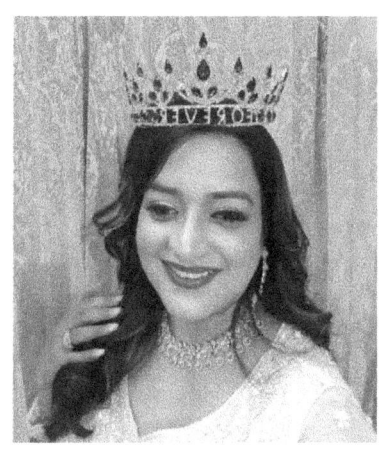

Victory for KawaljeetKauras She Clinches MrsAmritsar 2024 Title at City Finale

hindustan express

It's pouring love, blessings, and heartfelt wishes for the newly crowned Forever Mrs India, Kawaljeet, who became MrsAmritsar after her stunning victory at the City Finale of the 4th Season of Forever Miss India. The event, held from September 6th to 8th, 2024 In PAN India, was a celebration of talent, grace, and empowerment. Kawaljeetis now gearing up for the highly anticipated Grand Finale, which will take place in December 2024 in Jaipur, Rajasthan. Kawaljeet's journey to the City crown has been nothing short of remarkable. Throughout the talent rounds, she showcased her exceptional qualities, radiant personality, and unwavering dedication to making a positive impact in her community. With each step she took,

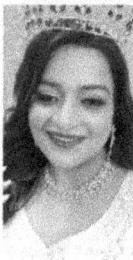

KawaljeetKaur left an indelible mark, capturing the hearts of judges, fellow contestants, and the audience alike. KawaljeetKaur, currently serving in a government position, has been named Mrs Amritsar City 2024. Passionate about personal growth and empowerment, Kaur aspires to become a Women Empowerment Coach. "Winning this title is a significant milestone," Kaur said. "My goal is to inspire women to see themselves as the creators of their own lives and to help them achieve their dreams through self-belief and action. I want to empower every woman to realize her potential and become the version of herself she aspires to be." The Forever Mrs India pageant celebrates the essence of womanhood, emphasizing inner beauty, strength, and global empowerment. Now an international platform, Forever Star India has already organized three successful seasons, and this 4th season is shaping up to be even more spectacular. The Grand Finale in December will be a grand celebration of talent and grace, setting the stage for an unforgettable conclusion to this incredible journey.

I have been crowned as "**Forever Star Mrs Punjab 2024**" (State Winner) too.

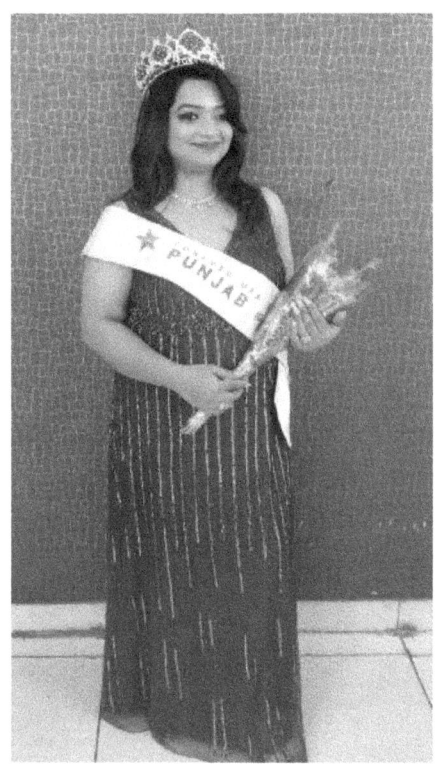

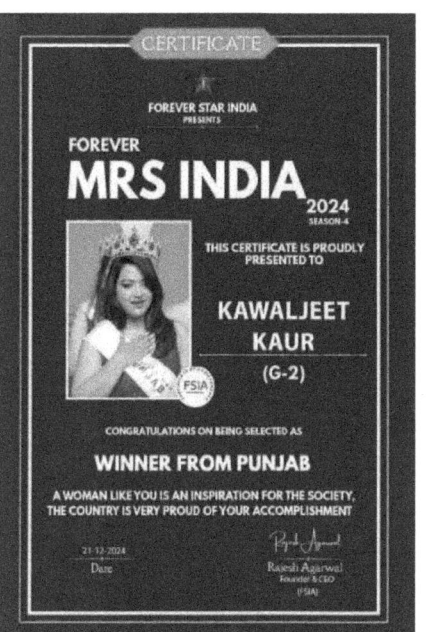

CERTIFICATE

FOREVER STAR INDIA PRESENTS

FOREVER MRS INDIA 2024
SEASON-4

THIS CERTIFICATE IS PROUDLY PRESENTED TO

KAWALJEET KAUR
(G-2)

CONGRATULATIONS ON BEING SELECTED AS

WINNER FROM PUNJAB

A WOMAN LIKE YOU IS AN INSPIRATION FOR THE SOCIETY, THE COUNTRY IS VERY PROUD OF YOUR ACCOMPLISHMENT

21-12-2024
Date

Rajesh Agarwal
Founder & CEO
(FSIA)

FOREVER STAR INDIA

Forever Mrs India 2024

Dear Kawaljeet Kaur,

Congratulations on Winning Forever Mrs India Punjab (G-2) 2024!

On behalf of the entire Forever Star India family, we would like to extend our heartfelt congratulations to you for being crowned Forever Mrs India Punjab (G-2) 2024! This prestigious title is a testament to your hard work, dedication, and immense talent. Your beauty, grace, and strength have truly shone through, and we are incredibly proud to have you represent Forever Star India with such poise and excellence.

Your victory is not just a personal achievement but an inspiration to countless women who dream of making their mark in the world. You have proven that with passion and perseverance, anything is possible. As you embark on this exciting new chapter of your journey, we have no doubt that you will continue to inspire and achieve great things.

Once again, congratulations on your well-deserved success. We wish you all the best in your future endeavors and look forward to supporting you in all your upcoming ventures.

21-Dec-24
Date

Rajesh Agarwal
CEO & Founder
(FSIA)

72-77, G1, Sadguru Apartments2, Gyan Vihar, Nirman Nagar
Jaipur, Rajasthan, 302019

I was blessed to walk the ramp as a "**Runway model**" in "**Forever Fashion Week**", World's First and Biggest Fashion Week Series by "**SHIE LOBO**" a famous show director and Runway choreographer.

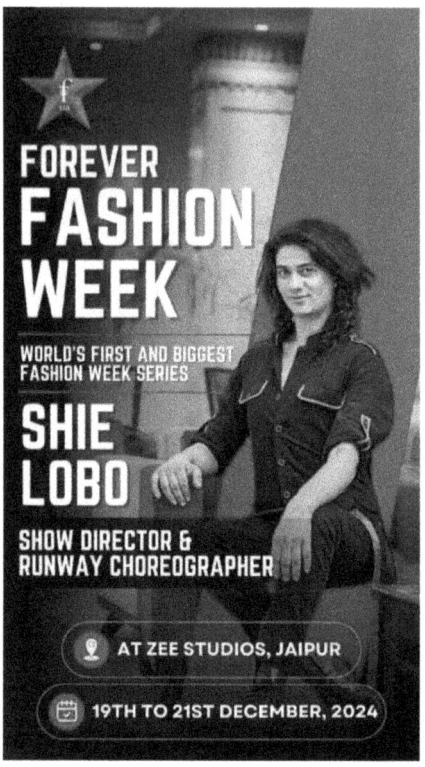 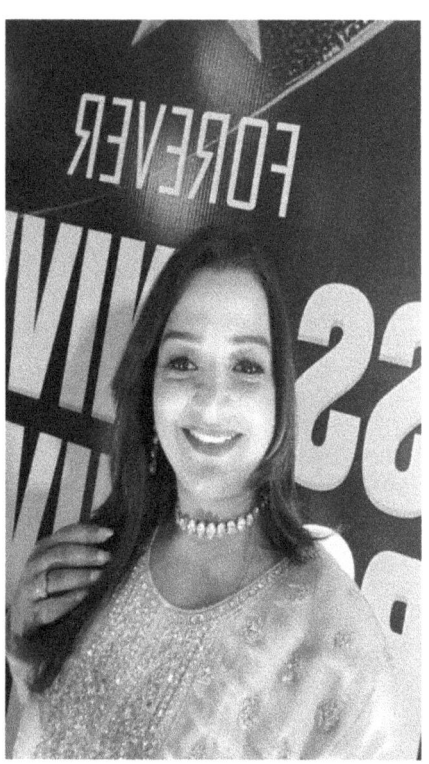

I have been awarded as the **"Best Inspiring Women"** from Punjab by a bollywood celebrity **Mr.Rahul Dev** hosted by **"Forever Star India Awards"**.

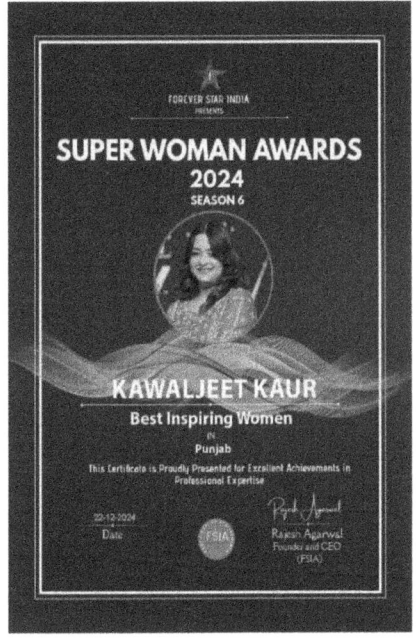

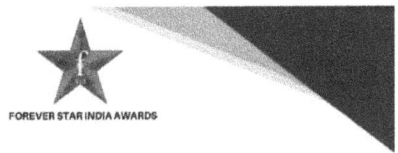

Certificate of Excellence

Dear Kawaljeet Kaur,

We are pleased to inform you that you have been selected as an awardee for the Super Woman Awards 2024 in the Best Inspiring Women From Punjab. This prestigious recognition highlights your dedication, hard work, and outstanding achievements in the business industry.

You are now authorized to proudly display this certificate, which reflects your success and your significant contributions to the field. Your recognition by the esteemed Rahul Dev and the Super Woman Awards is a testament to your leadership, vision, and commitment to excellence.

As part of this achievement, you can now use the official certificate for marketing, promotion, and professional representation, showcasing your excellence in the industry.

We congratulate you once again for this remarkable accomplishment and wish you continued success in your future endeavors.

Thank you,

22-Dec-24
Date

Rajesh Agarwal
CEO & Founder
(FSIA)

72-77, G1, Sadguru Apartments2, Gyan Vihar, Nirman Nagar
Jaipur, Rajasthan, 302019

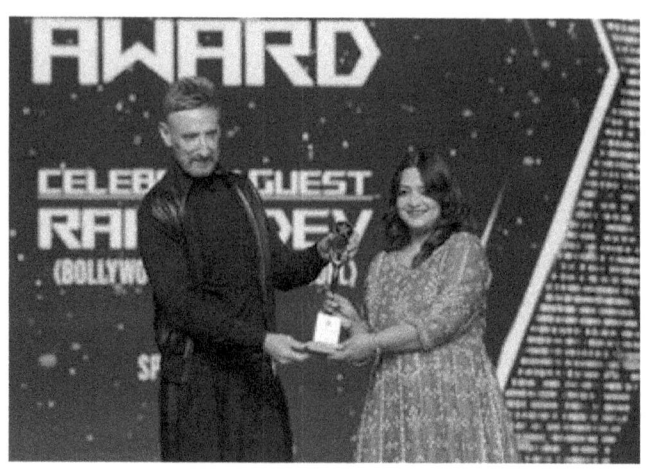

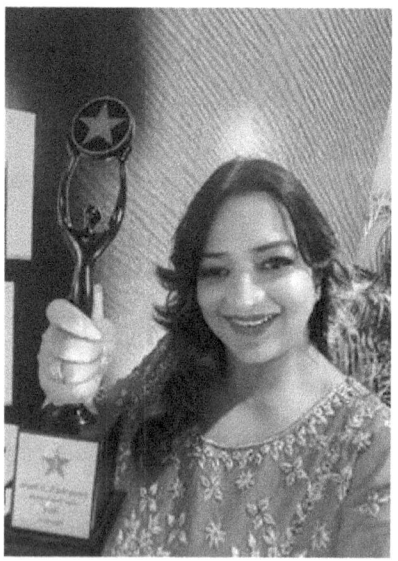

I have been awarded the **"City Excellence Award/25"** for my achievements.

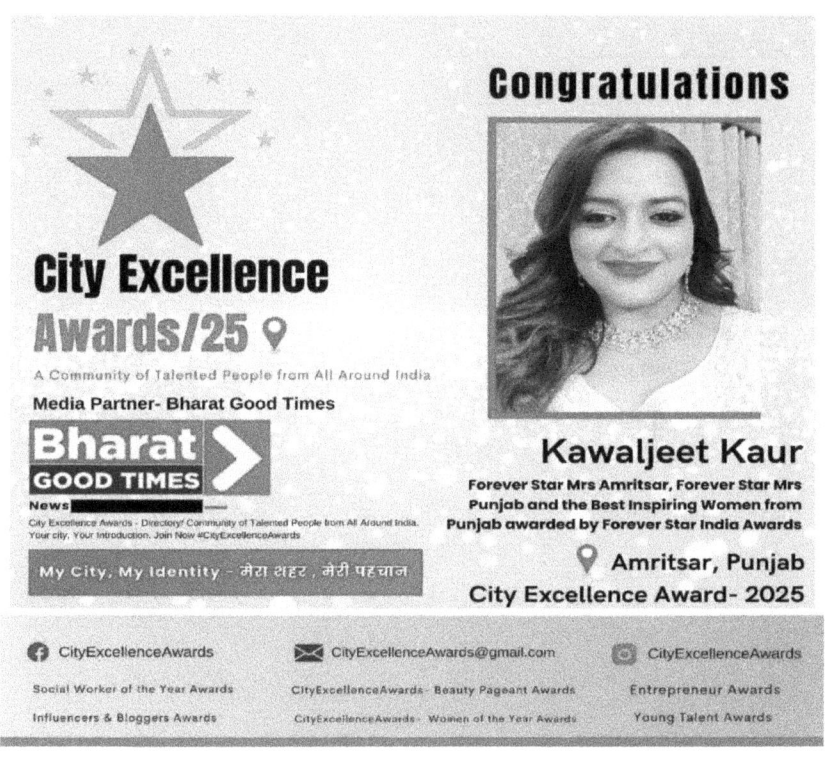

I have been on the cover page of "**Femmetimes Women Magazine**" January 2025 edition with an article on my journey.

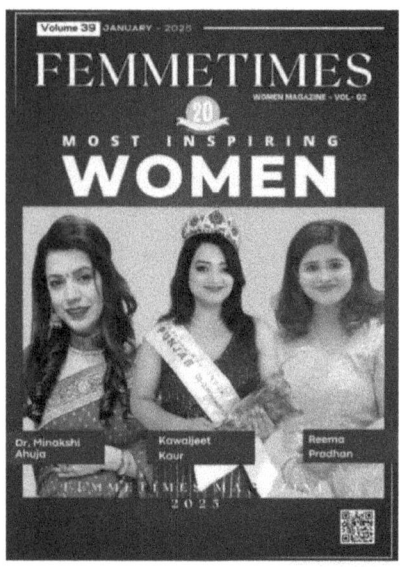

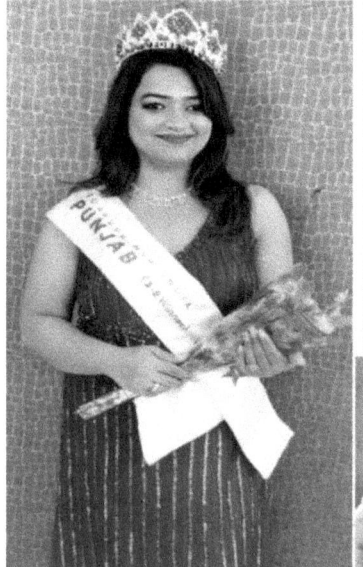

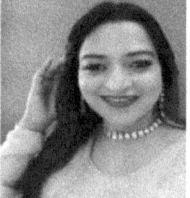

MOST INSPIRING WOMAN GLAM ICON-2025

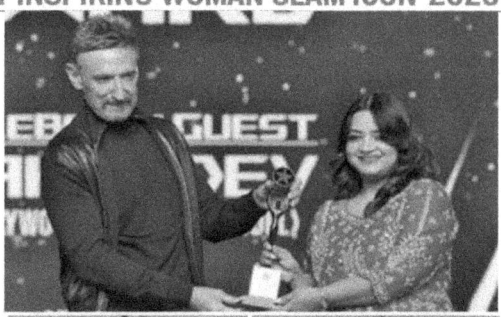

Her journey led her to the world of pageantry, where she not only broke free from the limiting beliefs that had once held her back but also emerged as a symbol of empowerment and strength. Kawaljeet proved to herself and others that success is not about following conventional paths, but about breaking barriers and embracing challenges. Through hard work, self-discipline, and a positive mindset, she achieved great milestones, winning titles like Forever Star Mrs. Amritsar and Forever Star Mrs. Punjab. Her accomplishments reflect a deep commitment to self-growth and a desire to inspire other women to rise above their circumstances. Looking ahead, Kawaljeet aims to further her impact by becoming a dedicated Women Empowerment Coach. As one of the most inspiring women from Punjab, her journey exemplifies how determination and resilience can transform lives. She dreams of mentoring women to not only overcome their challenges but to thrive in their personal and professional lives, Kawaljeet's ability to break through barriers and redefine success makes her a beacon of hope and empowerment.

This exceptional woman has the power to inspire and mentor others, offering guidance, motivation, and actionable strategies to help women unlock their true potential. She is ready to serve not just as an inspiration but as a coach, mentor, and guide to women seeking to overcome adversity and achieve their dreams.

For mentorship or to connect with Kawaljeet Kaur, she can be reached via email at kaurkawaljit8299@gmail.com or gurpreetsingh.alniche@gmail.com

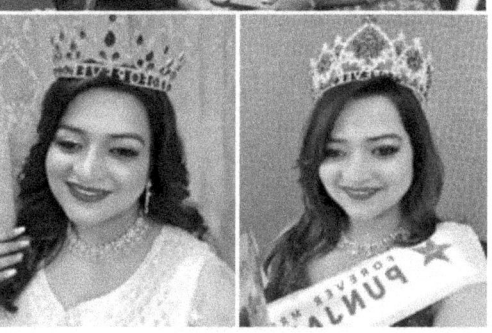

SOME Q AND A WITH KAWALJEET KAUR:

Q. What motivated you to pursue pageantry alongside your government job?

■ **Kawaljeet Kaur:** "Breaking the glass ceiling of my limiting beliefs was my biggest motivation. For a long time, I struggled with mental blockages that made me doubt my abilities. Pageantry provided the perfect platform to challenge myself, proving to myself and others that I could excel even in an unfamiliar domain. It was not about modelling or fame—it was about breaking barriers and proving that with determination, I could achieve what once seemed impossible."

Q. How do you balance your career and your passion for modelling and pageantry?

■ **Kawaljeet Kaur:** "Interestingly, pageantry and modelling have never been my passion. My real passion lies in challenging my limits and growing as a person. When the opportunity arose, I treated it as a chance to push beyond my comfort zone. I balanced my government job and pageantry by staying focused on my priorities and managing time effectively. Ultimately, the experience enriched me and led to success as a city and state winner, reinforcing my belief in continuous self-improvement."

Q. What message do you have for women aspiring to break stereotypes?

■ **Kawaljeet Kaur:** "Questioning and breaking stereotypes is the first step toward self-discovery. I encourage every woman to challenge societal norms and embrace the journey of personal growth. Focus on becoming your best version—invest in yourself, your dreams, and your mindset. Breaking stereotypes isn't just about defying others' expectations; it's about realizing your potential and living a life true to yourself."

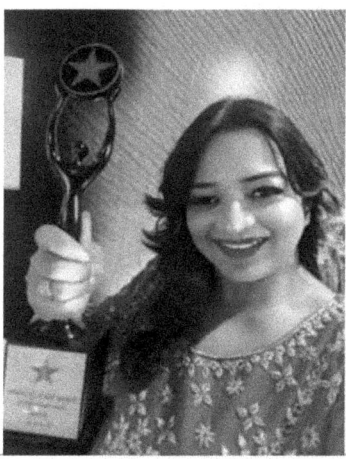

The article on my journey of life and my achievements is published in the famous **"Lifestyle"** magazine edition of March' 2025.

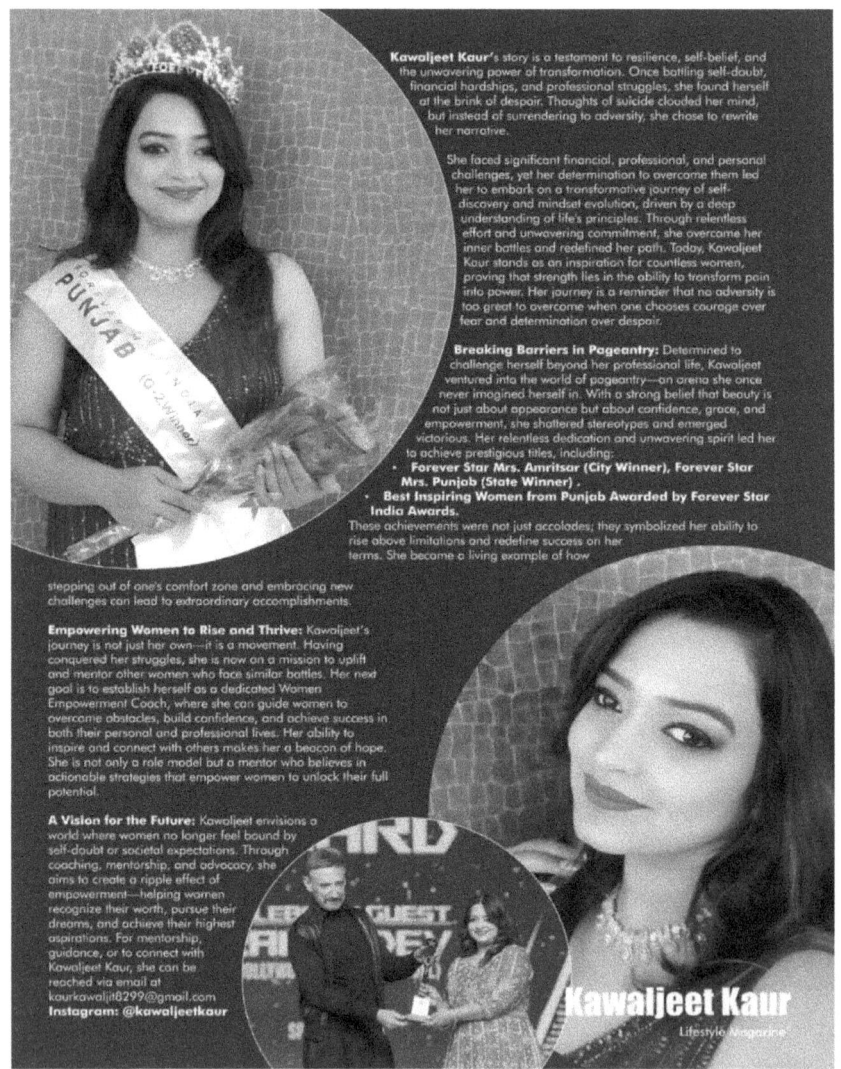

Acknowledgements

I bow before all the divine powers of this universe with a grateful heart that guided, supported, and lined up everything to manifest my dream into reality through this book and making me step into this new role of being an "AUTHOR."

Hi, my name is Kawaljeet Kaur, the author of this book and I have spent more than half a decade finding the answers to those unlimited questions about life I was surrounded with, just like you. Throughout this journey, I have learned various lessons, techniques and the laws of the universe to make my life better.I have worked on transforming myself from within, and here I am to help you out by answering those endless questions about life and yourself and helping you transform yourself to be your better version and achieve your dreams.

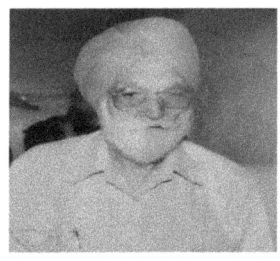 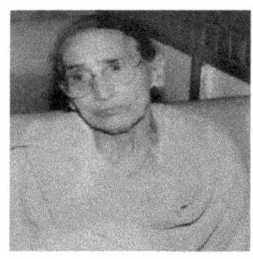

Late S.Harchand Singh   Late.Smt.Satnam Kaur
   (Nana Papa)   (Nani Maa)

I am grateful to my grandparents Late. S.Sawran Singh and Late. Smt.Bachan Kaur for being my grandparents and showering their love and blessings. I am grateful to my maternal grandparents Late S.Harchand Singh and Late.Smt.Satnam Kaur for upbringing me and my siblings with all the love, care and support when my parents were busy in earning money to give me and my brothers a beautiful and a comfortable life.

Thank you, Thank you, Thank you.

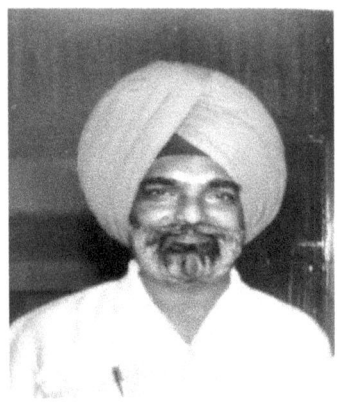
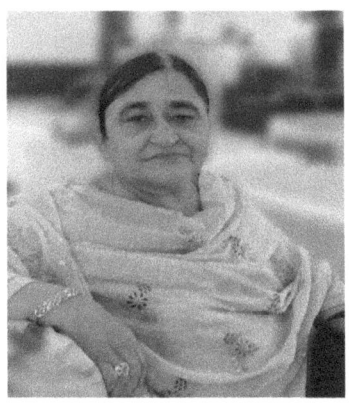

Late.S.Hardyal Singh   Mrs. Harjit Kaur
(my father)   (my mother)

I dedicate this book in the loving memory of my father, the late S.Hardyal Singh, who would always be an inseparable part of my life and whose upbringing, values, love, and dreams pushed me to this moment of my life and my loving mom, Mrs.Harjit Kaur, who is a living legend for me and because of whose love, support and guidance I am who I am.I truly feel beyond blessed to have you both as my parents.

Thank you, Thank you, Thank you.

I dedicate this book to the most loving and angelic soul, "Manav," my nephew, for giving me the moments to experience that unconditional love, happiness, joy and laughter.

Thank you, Thank you, Thank you.

I owe this book to my personal coach, Miss. Gazal Gupta, who has worked endlessly with all her dedication, love and support in helping me transform and become my better version.

Thank you, Thank you, Thank you.

I owe this book to all other mentors, namely Mrs. Anjana Reetoria, Mr.Bob Proctor, Dr. Joe Dispenza, Mr.Mitesh Khatri, Coach BSR and many more, who helped me in my journey of transformation through their seminars, webinars, sessions, videos and books. I am truly thankful for the abundance of knowledge that I received from them that helped me transform my life and be a better version of myself.

Thank you, Thank you, Thank you.

I am grateful to the Late S.Santokh Singh Bhamra, Late Smt.Mans Kaur Bhamra, S.Sarbjit Singh, Mrs.Gursharanjeet Kaur, S.Gurtejinder Singh, Mrs.Jagriti Ranga, Dr.Rajinder Singh, S.Davinder Singh for supporting me in this journey in every possible way.

Thank you, Thank you, Thank you.

Thanks to the love of my life, my life partner S.Gurpreet Singh, whose love and support brought me to this moment of my life.

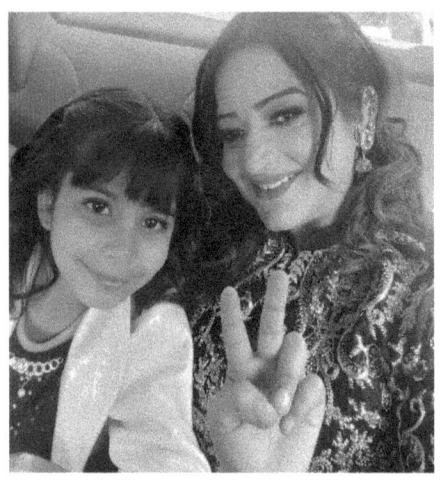

Me with my Daughter "JAZZLEEN"

I am truly grateful for the driving force of my life, my daughter "Jazzleen," as this book would be a lifelong gift for her.

I am grateful for all those loving, kind and supportive people around me in my professional life who have supported me with all their positivity, encouragement and appreciation in turning my dream into reality.

Thank you, Thank you, Thank you.

My heartfelt thanks to the publishers of this book, the "BlueRose Publishers" team, for all their support, guidance and help in bringing my vision into reality by publishing my book.

Thank you, Thank you, Thank you.

Thank you, Thank you, Thank you to my ancestors, angels and every soul I have ever met that helped me, motivated me, inspired me, supported me in any way in this lifetime. The ones I might have forgotten by now.

Thank you, Thank you, Thank you to every reader of my book for trusting me to help you transform your life for the better.

Thank you, Thank you, Thank you to all the divine powers of the universe for this wonderful experience of my life.

Contents

What is Life? 1

We are Creators 6

Powers of our Mind 22

Gratitude is the Key 43

The 2 ways to Elevated Emotions 55

Script your life 59

Visualization 65

Vision Boards 72

Richness of Health 77

Richness of Relationships 86

Richness of Money 92

Richness of Career 105

What is Life?

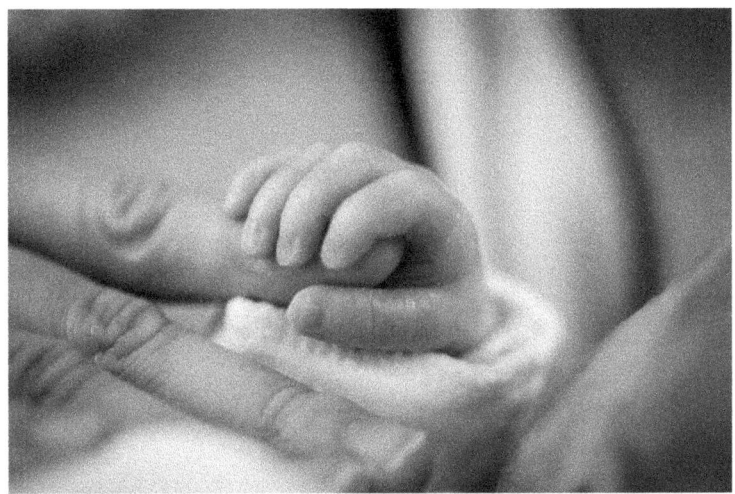

Let's connect with each other over a simple and very basic question.

"What is life according to you?" Take a pause and think about it.

What do you think life is?

Are you the one who thinks that life is predestined? Everything is already written. Your bad days, your struggles, your health issues, your relationship issues-everything is already written in your destiny and there is nothing you can do with it. Are you the one who feels that others are more intelligent, more successful, more lucky or extraordinary than you and you are just an ordinary one? Do you wish to be as intelligent, successful and lucky as other people? Do you feel that another person has a better destiny than yours? Do you feel that you were born to experience struggles in life? If the answer to the above question is "yes," then I assure you that by the time you finish reading this book, your perspective towards yourself and your life will be completely changed and you will be able to understand how powerful and special you are and how you yourself design your life, *"consciously or unconsciously."*

Now, if you ask me what life is, I would answer you in one sentence:

"Life is what you make it."

Yes, your life is what you make it. It is exactly what you choose to make it.

Your life is the sum total of all the choices you have made in each moment in every aspect of your life and these choices include what you allow yourself to feed your mind with, what you speak, what you read, and what you see. These all form your various beliefs and your life is then governed by these beliefs.

Let's dive deeper into this.

Like you, I too, at some point in my life, thought that there was some Supreme Power who had already written my good days, my bad days and my struggles-the one who had already sketched my life. Life was really hard those days. Even though I am a highly qualified person who did a Masters in Law, the time came when I just wanted to end up with everything (my life), and at that exact moment, I realized that my academic certificates and qualifications were not enough for me to live a happy, prosperous and abundant life. You too might have faced such situations and circumstances in your life when you too felt that there was much more we needed to know and learn about life apart from our formal education in schools and colleges. When I was flooded with all those negative thoughts about ending up with my life, I came across a quote on my phone. A quote that says, "**Your life is what you make it.**" And the words just blew my mind. How is this possible? I questioned myself, "What are these words trying to convey?" I never wanted my life to be at this point.I read this statement over and over again. I never wanted to experience these struggles in my life. My mind was then flooded with more such questions, like "How are some people so happy?" "How are some people so rich?" "How are successful people so successful?" "How do they have such loving relationships?" as I was not enjoying any of these. *I was the one who felt like giving up on life.*

Then what? My search for these answers started. Slowly and gradually, I came to know about the various successful people who experienced tremendous success in every area of life. Now my next question was, "How are they able to do it?" as I was feeling helpless in every aspect of my life and in today's digital world, finding an answer to our questions (no matter how confusing or challenging the question is) is just a click away. It started my journey of personal development. My curiosity about the subject forced me to dive deeper and deeper, challenging what I was learning and then practicing and experiencing the results. And now, after a decade of my journey of personal development, a day came when I felt a strong impulse to share my experience, my knowledge, my wisdom and my learnings with the world by writing the book with the intention of helping others. This book would definitely help in changing an unlimited number of lives and would bring more love, abundance, prosperity, health, wealth, happiness and anything you ever dreamed of; you are capable enough to achieve it.

The way you perceive life, life will perceive you in the same way. If you feel life is not good, it will not give you anything good, but if you feel life is good or beautiful, it will gift you with all such beautiful and wonderful experiences to cherish. It all depends on how you perceive life. Just like a glass of water that is half full and half empty, if you ask someone what they think of looking at the glass, one will say that it is half empty and the other might say that it is half full. So this is only your perspective on looking at the things that seem to be positive or negative to you. The same half filled glass seems to be half empty to someone, and the other half-empty glass seems to be half-filled to another. So, the same situation or the same experience can have different perspectives for different people, and here is where the whole trick lies. Life is nothing but your perspective or mindset to view, analyze and understand things. If you take life positively and learn even in the worst of your times, life is a great teacher, but if you take it negatively, life is a struggle; it's a hell.

Do you know something? We all have the tendency to cry, criticize, crib and blame others for little things, but we always forget to look inside us and check what thoughts we have, what attitude we possess and what self talk we do with ourselves, as these all frame our external world. We always forget these.

In my journey of personal development, the more I worked on my thoughts, the more I learned. I learned that instead of responding, I always reacted to every situation. Instead of being kind to others, I was filled with grudges and anger towards them. Instead of being loving to others, I was harsh to them with my words. Instead of using positive self-talk, I was relying on negative self-talk. Then what could I expect as a result? It was exactly what I was giving out that was coming back to me.

In the upcoming pages, we will dive deep into "How our lives are shaped?" And if at any moment you feel that something is wrong in any aspect of your life, you could definitely change it in your favor, as it is rightly said, "Your life is what you make it ." I'm repeating this statement because I want you to understand that ONLY AND ONLY **"YOU"** ARE THE CREATOR AND THE MASTER OF YOUR LIFE AND ONLY **"YOU"** CAN CHANGE YOUR LIFE STORY AT ANY MOMENT, **ONCE YOU DECIDE FOR IT.**

"Life is what we make it, always has been, always will be."

-Grandma Moses
(A folk artist)

We are Creators

"Your thoughts and feelings create your life. It will always be that way. Guaranteed"

-Lisa Nicholas
(Motivational Speaker and Author)

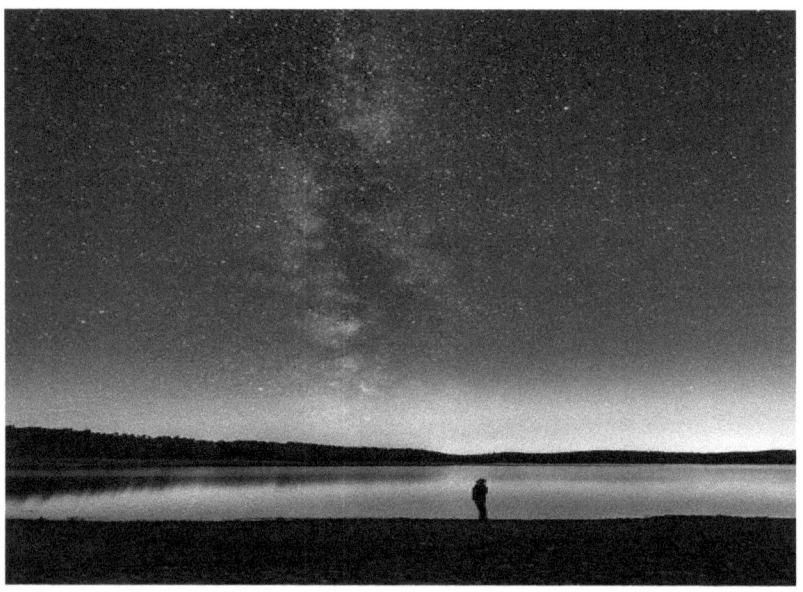

Yes, we are all creators of our lives with our thoughts, words, beliefs and actions. Now your next question would be, "How?" How are we the creators of our lives?

Read carefully and try to understand what is being shared now.

Everything in this world is "ENERGY." Everything that exists is made up of energy in some form, as matter is an illusion of energy and light. It's not physical. Atoms are the basic building blocks for all matter, which are further made up of electrons, protons and neutrons and that is energy, not substance. We humans too are all fundamentally "AN ENERGY." Human cells are made up of multiple atoms. Everything in the universe is made up of atoms. What differentiates us from other things is the density of the atoms and their vibrational frequency. Our body is a molecular structure consisting of trillions of cells vibrating at very high speed. We humans are an organization of energy with different degrees of vibration based on what we think, feel, speak and do. The world around us is full of energy, vibrations and frequencies.

All objects are vibrating. Earth and stars are vibrating. Nothing is solid. Even our materialistic goals, such as a car, bungalow or phone, everything is energy. Everything is energy and vibration. No energy can ever be lost. It can only change its form. Even water and glass are energy. The speed at which it is vibrating is different. We are all energy fields wherever we go. We are broadcasting energy. And so, we are all connected, as we are all energy.

Einstein's famous equation

$E = MC^2$

says that energy and mass are two forms of the same thing and can be converted into each other. Hence, all matter contains energy. Every atom, particle and molecule is in a constant state of vibration. All things, even all objects, are solid and still made from energy at a very basic level. Everything is moving, vibrating and full of energy.

> *"This whole world boils down to one word "energy." It's free and you can use it for you or against you, but it must be used."*
>
> *-John roger*
> *(American Author and Public Speaker)*

Science says that energy is never created nor destroyed ; rather, it can only change its form.

Let's understand it better with the help of an example:

Suppose there is cold water. If it is kept in a refrigerator to freeze, it will turn into ice and if the same water is kept on fire and boiled, its form will change and the water will turn into steam. Energy only changes its form. It can never be created nor destroyed.

We are all spiritual beings and spirit never dies. It could only take rebirth. We are spirit and spirit is energy.

"How do thoughts and words affect our lives? "

EVERYTHING VIBRATES, NOTHING RESTS

Energy has a vibration and vibration has a frequency. Energy vibrates at a certain frequency. If you look at our human body through a microscope, you will find that nothing is static. It is not still. Everything vibrates. Everything in the universe, from the smallest atom to the largest galaxy, is in a continuous state of motion and energy. We humans are all vibrating beings with our own unique frequencies depending on our thoughts, emotions, beliefs and actions that affect our vibrations and ultimately affect our reality. This energy vibrates at a different rate or frequency depending on its nature and state. We attract what we are in harmony with.

Remember the law that we all studied in our 9th and 10th grades?

"LIKE ATTRACTS LIKE"

This is another cosmic law. You will always attract to yourself what corresponds to your dominant thoughts. You attract into your life what you are. If you have more loving, kind and happy thoughts, you will attract such people around you. We are all magnets and we attract what we are. People of similar thoughts are attracted towards each other. That's why it is said, "Birds of the same feather flock together." This law is always operating, whether you are conscious of it or not.

As we are all energy, the thoughts we think generate emotions and feelings in our bodies and the words that we use give pictures to our minds. When we use negative words and think negative thoughts, we then start transmitting a negative signal or energy into the universe. On the other hand, when we use positive words, we send positive energy to the universe with our feelings. Look at the results of your life and your results show which vibrations you are on. Our vibrations decide what we attract in our lives. Our vibrations decide what we are in harmony with. To change results, change your vibrations.

The laws of the universe follow you everywhere, whether you believe them or not. They are precise and clear. In the same way, the law of gravity works. If anything is to be thrown, it would not go towards the sky, rather; it would be pulled down to the earth. An apple from a tree falls on earth; it never goes to the sky. It's all due to the law of gravity. Whether you believe it or not, these laws are always there and these laws are always working. When you start believing in the laws of the universe, you start creating the life you want.

HOW DOES ENERGY AFFECT OUR LIVES?

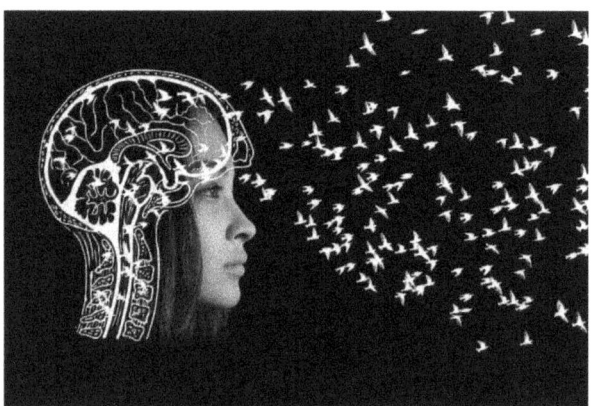

Our thoughts and feelings generate vibrations that ripple out into the universe. Vibration is the law of the universe. We all think in terms of frequencies. The thoughts we are thinking and the emotions we are feeling are producing results in our lives. We can only choose which frequency to operate on. The universe only responds to our vibration. It always gives us exactly what we need to live our lives aligned with the vibration and frequency we are on. The only thing you have to focus on is keeping your vibrations high. It could be through prayer, meditation, or dancing. Anything that you love doing will make you vibe high. Let's say if you want to be rich and successful in life, you cannot manifest it with the thoughts that I am not good enough, I can never be successful, I am poor because the words you are speaking and emotions you are feeling are just the lack of being successful and rich and it can only attract to you the people, situations and circumstances that would prove to you that you are definitely not good enough, you can never be successful or you are poor for sure, as this is what the law of vibration would bring back to you.

Everything is energy, which means airplanes, helicopters and money are energy. Now, if you want more money in your life, you cannot attract it by continuously feeling a lack of it. Feeling the lack of money in your life means you are tuning or attracting those situations and circumstances in your life where you would experience more of a lack of money. It's just like a radio. When you want to listen to 104.8 FM, you would tune the radio to that frequency and the song that would be playing there would be audible to you. In the same way, if you want to listen to 94.2 FM, you will tune your radio to that frequency and hear the song that is being played.

If you start feeling that you are already living a life of prosperity and abundance and you emit that energy of being abundant and prosperous with your words, feelings and actions, you will attract such people, situations, circumstances and events into your life that would make you prosperous and abundant. You can only attract into your life those that are in vibrational harmony with you. You must see yourself living with your desires fulfilled and hold on to that image in your mind. Believe that it's going to come and that will attract everything to you to turn your desire into reality.

Many times, you must have noticed that when something goes wrong at the beginning of the day, a series of negative situations continue the whole day. It's because once you get into low vibrations, you attract more of such negative or low vibrational incidents in your life. The other days, when something positive or great happens to you in the morning, your whole day is filled with excitement, happiness, and joy. It's all due to the energy you have. When you emit negative energy into the universe, the same energy, be it in the form of people, situations, or circumstances, is attracted back to you in your life. On the other hand, when you give positive energy to the universe, you attract positive people, situations, and circumstances in your life. That's why we have heard many such stories where one incident went wrong and the chain of wrong incidents in someone's life starts. The example goes otherwise too. There are people who experience one win, and then the chain of good incidents just continues. It's all because the one negative incident succeeded in lowering the vibrations and attracted more negative experiences, while in the other case, one positive experience pulled the person towards other good experiences because the thought became so positive and uplifting.

"If you want to find the secrets of the universe, think in terms of energy, frequency and vibration."

-Nikola Tesla
(An American inventor and an electrical engineer)

THE SCIENCE OF QUANTUM PHYSICS

Quantum physics is the study of matter and energy. The science of quantum physics says that nothing is reality until you observe it with your thoughts and energy. Everything that exists in the quantum field, be it your better version, your better life, or your luxurious lifestyle, always exists, but you can only experience what you are observing through your thoughts. The one you are experiencing now is the one you observed through your thoughts and energy.

Let's make it more clear with the following example:

At any given time, all the songs that have ever been created exist, but you cannot listen to all the songs at the same time. It would be overstimulating and wouldn't give you any enjoyment. Now, suppose you feel like listening to a piece of music. You would choose that song that would meet your preferences, like what mood you are in. Do you want to listen to a sad song or a dancing number? Whatever would be your preferences, you would choose the song accordingly.

Now, when you play your preferred song and start listening to it, it is in your physical reality. You are now experiencing listening to your preferred song through your five senses. Now, just think: when you are listening to this particular song of your choice, does that mean there is no other song? No, there are millions and millions of songs that exist, but you called upon this song in your physical reality. In the same way, the life you are living now is the life you have summoned through your thoughts and if you want to experience a better life, start focusing on better and more positive thoughts to summon them in your life so that you can experience it with your five senses. If you want to change your life, you can change your life trajectory. It's possible, as it also exists in quantum potential.

You must be wondering that you want health, wealth, happiness and success in your life and why they're not showing up in your life. The answer is that most of you are thinking about what you don't have and what you don't want and you end up attracting all that in your life that you don't want. Instantly focus all your energy on what you want to manifest in your life. Focus all your energy on being grateful for what you have now. The thing to understand is that we have all been programmed since childhood to experience a lack of money, lack of confidence, lack of intelligence, lack of happiness, support, love and much more. We are programmed this way now. We are never taught in school about life. How do we live a beautiful life? We are never taught about money and when, after spending 12 to 15 years of our formal education, we come out of schools and colleges completing our education, facing life becomes such a big challenge that some do commit suicide, some spoil their lives with other unhealthy activities, some struggle with their mental and physical health and some struggle in other spheres of life. No one ever taught us how to take charge of our lives.

To attract the success and richness you want to experience in your life, you first must feel that you are successful and rich in this moment. You must feel the emotions of being rich and successful right now. Create a mental picture of you being rich and successful. Feeling does not need materialistic things before you. You can feel any emotion at any time, imagining the worst or the best of your life. You must imagine your body language, your expressions, your attitude and your feelings if you become rich and successful. You have to live that role and when you do it on a consistent basis, you are emitting a strong signal in the universe in the form of energy and vibrations that you are that person and then the magic happens and boom, you will start attracting those people, situations and circumstances into your life that would help you become that successful and rich version of yourself.

"Everything is energy and that's all there is to it. Match the frequency of the reality you want and you cannot help but get that reality. It can be no other way. This is not philosophy. This is physics."

-Albert Einstein
(A physicist and a Noble Prize winner in physics)

TAKE 100% RESPONSIBILITY OF YOUR LIFE.

Nothing and no one are to blame. It was your thoughts, emotions and feelings that matched the frequency of any negative situation or circumstance and thus attracted such circumstances and people into your life. To change the circumstances, just start focusing on the good in your life.

"The only way we can change our lives is to change our energy- to change the electromagnetic field we are constantly broadcasting. In other words, to change our state of being, we have to change how we think and how we feel."

-Dr. Joe Dispenza
(New York Times Bestseller Author, Researcher and Lecturer)

By aligning your thoughts, emotions and actions with your desires, you can attract anything you desire. You must have a sincere desire to achieve anything that you want in life. There must be a fire in your desire and imagine the emotions of your desire being fulfilled.

You need not work for your problems once you understand these laws. You need to work on getting to higher vibrations. Negativity can only affect you if you are on the same frequency. So be the energy you want to attract into your life.

You are not the victim of any circumstance, no matter how bad it is. Rather, you are the story writer, the director and of course, the actor of your own life once you decide to make it. Nothing on this earth can stop you from achieving your dreams. The barriers that we all usually experience are just the barriers of our own limitations in our minds.

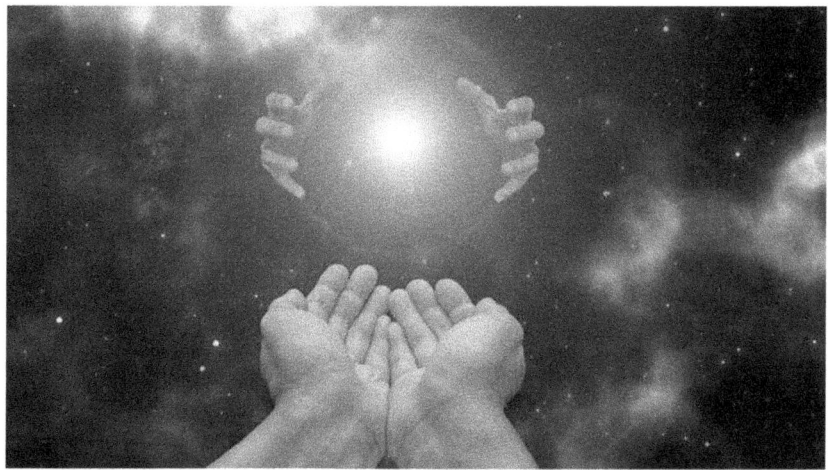

UNIVERSE ONLY RESPONDS TO YOUR VIBRATIONS

The universe only responds to your vibration. There are no accidents or coincidences in this world. There are synchronicities. Everything is co-created. Anything and everything you experience is a manifestation of where your energy is focused.

Once you start understanding and mastering your thoughts and feelings, you become the creator of your own reality. You then learn how to use your power to create the life you want. Your emotions and your feelings are a great signal to understand what vibrations you are in. If you are feeling the emotions of love, peace, joy, happiness and gratitude, you are in high vibrations. If you are feeling angry, sad, disheartened or jealous, you are feeling low vibrational emotions.

ENERGY IS CONTAGIOUS

Energy is contagious. Be conscious of your surroundings and the people you hang out with because we are all energy and energy is contagious. It is rightly said that if you hang out with the five millionaires, you will be the sixth one and if you hang out with the five idiots, you will be the sixth one because the thoughts, the words and the actions define our energy, in which energy we are.

Our emotions are energy. To keep your emotions elevated, you must choose the right kind of people to be around, as you will be influenced by their energy. Don't sit among general people rather; spend more time among those people like whom you want to become, as energy is contagious.

EMOTIONAL CONTAGION

The other scientific reason behind choosing the right people to be around is that we all have mirror neurons in dispersed areas of our brain and these mirror neurons are always paying attention to other people's emotional states. The moment they identify the emotional state of other people, they mirror it and we feel it and it's called emotional contagion. That's why negative emotions or low vibrations like anger, stress and anxiety could be contagious. You must have felt that when someone comes to you stressed, you feel it too. Similarly, it works for positive emotions too. If you are around happy and joyful people, you will catch those vibrations. That's why it is important to choose your association, the people you hang out with "wisely."

ENERGY NEVER LIES

Many times, we feel stuck in our lives. It is nothing but blocked energy inside us that wants to move. When these stuck emotions cause stress or anxiety, it's the energy asking you to help it move. In other words, whenever you feel that you are stuck in your life, try to spend some time in the energy of a person who is happy and joyful. You would start feeling better in some time.

It is our energy in the room first that introduces us to others, even before we say anything. Many times, when we are with someone, we feel sad, uncomfortable, or even drained out without any communication with that person. That is the energy telling you to save yourself. Don't deny the energy or vibes you feel about certain people or situations. If it's not making you feel right, it's not right because energy never lies. That is a sign that we may or may not spend much time. Many times, we meet such people that their energy feels so familiar to us that we feel that we have already met them. It's all about energy.

Make a list of the things that could help you shift your energy instantly. It could be music, meditation, dancing, reading something uplifting, remembering those funny moments, watching comedy scenes, thinking of happy moments, remembering beautiful memories or spending time in nature. Do anything that uplifts your energy and makes you feel happier.

So, learn to protect your energy from people who do not make you feel happy, and joyful in life. To attract happiness and joy into your life, you first must emit those vibrations.

You don't have to kill your problems or create opportunities; you just have to change your frequency and you will then attract opportunities and the right people into your life.

Here are some key points you could take care of to protect vibes:

1. Never compare yourself with anyone.//
2. Work on your fears.
3. Please yourself instead of others.
4. Stay away from those people who drain your energy.
5. Be kind to yourself and others with your actions and your words.
6. Let go of all those things you just cannot control.
7. No gossip about others, as it lowers your vibrations.
8. Learn to say "No" to the things that do not feel right to you.
9. Do something that makes you feel more happy and joyful each day.

10. Spend time with yourself. Understand yourself.

Check out the results in your life. If you are continuously attracting problems in your life, it shows that you are on a low vibration and you can change it at any moment. Become what you want.

If you want love, be love.

If you want happiness, be happy.

If you want peace, be peaceful.

"You attract what you are and not what you want in your life." Yes, you attract into your life what you are and what you are includes your behaviors, beliefs and patterns, which have now become part of you. Let's study it more deeply to understand how our lives are framed in our next topic, "Powers of our Mind."

Powers of our Mind

Now the question is:

"Why are we humans special among all other living creatures on this planet?"

We humans are God's best creation. It's because only we humans are blessed with mental faculties like perception, willpower, memory, reason, intuition, intellect, and the powers of thinking, imagining and visualizing. These mental faculties make us so powerful that we can design our lives the way we want it to be. Our mind is a powerful weapon. It's a tool to harness success in every sphere of life.

Our mind is divided into two parts: the conscious mind and the subconscious mind. The conscious mind governs only 5% of our lives, whereas the subconscious mind governs 95% of our lives. The conscious mind helps us to take decisions. It helps us decide how to respond. However, our subconscious mind is a habit mind and it has unlimited power. The conscious mind has all five senses. It has free will and the ability to accept or reject any idea. It is the one who decides our level of vibration. Your feeling is nothing but the awareness of vibration. It's a thinking mind. The subconscious mind is the power center and it connects with all the knowledge of the universe. It has all the answers to every question of yours. The subconscious mind is also referred to as "the spirit."

You are alive. Blood is circulating in your body, your kidneys and lungs are functioning, your heart is beating and this is all doing its functions in an automatic mode. This is all controlled by your subconscious mind. The subconscious mind is your emotional mind.

Many times, we try to change our external world, but it seems all in vain. Our lives mirror before us, in our external world what all we have inside us and to change our lives and to get desired results, we first need to reprogram our subconscious mind with various techniques. Our subconscious mind holds the most power in shaping our reality and all our experiences, beliefs and memories that influence our behaviors, thoughts and actions.

If you are not experiencing what you want in your life, then there are some beliefs, memories and behavioral patterns that are stored in your subconscious mind and are showing up in your life in the form of your experiences. Look at your results your relationships, your career, and your life in every aspect. We are all attempting to change the results outside without changing what is inside us. It would be as foolish as standing before the mirror and trying to change the reflection in the mirror without changing our physical appearance. To experience love, peace, happiness, abundance and prosperity in your life, you first have to reprogram your subconscious mind with different techniques, which we will discuss in the upcoming pages.

Our subconscious mind is so powerful that it has all the answers to our questions. You can question yourself before going to sleep, like, "Who am I?" "What is my purpose on this planet?" "How can I contribute in this world?" Very soon, your subconscious mind will give you the answers to your every question. The situations or people in your life will somehow give you the answer to your questions. The subconscious mind is our inner mind and until and unless we work on our inner mind, we cannot experience any changes in our outer or external world. Our subconscious mind lives in the present moment, neither in the past nor in the future. It lives in "NOW." It does not differentiate between you imagining something or something truly happening in your reality. Whatever is impressed in the subconscious mind is expressed in our reality.

Do you understand why you are not able to live the life you want because your subconscious mind is programmed otherwise. We all have consciously or unconsciously programmed our subconscious mind and the struggles we face in our lives are all due to that programming. Whenever you encounter any of your wrong beliefs or limiting beliefs in any sphere of life, be it health, career, money or relationship, repeat to yourself, "I am free from this limiting belief from this moment onwards; I am free now; I am free; free forever."

There could be an unending list of our limiting beliefs. Few of them be like:

I always have to struggle to get something in life.

I am always late.

I cannot trust anyone.

It's hard to earn money.

Money comes with hard work.

Life is hard.

Life is a struggle.

Life is a series of ups and downs.

REPETITION or SELF HYPNOSIS

The good news is that our subconscious mind could be reprogrammed with repetition and self-hypnosis. When you repeat a particular thought again and again, it seeps into your subconscious mind and becomes your new way of thinking. Our subconscious mind accepts whatever is repeatedly said to it. To change your life in a positive way, you need to change the programming and give a new thought pattern to your subconscious mind.

Let's understand how our mind works. Our minds work at different frequencies. These are:

1. Beta: Awake, Normal Alert Consciousness

2. Alpha: Relaxed, Calm, Lucid, not thinking.

3. Theta: Deep relaxation and meditation, mental imagery.

4. Delta: Deep, Dreamless Sleep.

The above are the four different brainwaves and the most appropriate brainwave is the theta brainwave, in which we could reprogram our subconscious mind for our success. Theta is a brainwave when, if any command is given, it goes straight into our subconscious mind and we experience these brainwaves exactly 5 minutes before going to sleep and immediately after we wake up. Every night, 5 minutes before sleeping, turn over a specific request to your subconscious mind and experience the miracle of it happening in your life. You can do self-hypnosis and repetition too and this could be done immediately after you wake up and 5 minutes before you go to sleep.

Our brain in the first 7 years is operating in theta brain waves and is programmed with the words we heard from others, the actions and the behaviors we experienced around us. If we have experienced more disempowering words or attitudes from others, that results in limiting beliefs as we grow up. It works the other way around too. If in our childhood we experienced great conversations of love, abundance and prosperity among the people around us, our subconscious mind will work in our favor and will deliver us everything we want to experience in our lives.

THE TETRIS EFFECT

The "TETRIS EFFECT" says that the last thing you see before sleeping and the first thing you see after waking up get imprinted in your subconscious mind and at both these times, your subconscious mind is very open to suggestions. You can have a vision board before you with all the images of what you want to experience in your life. At both of these times, your brain goes through theta brain waves. Theta is a brainwave frequency that is associated with rapid programming and hypnosis and during these times we are entering the world of our subconscious mind. So, whatever command you give to your mind at both these important times of the day, your brain starts reprogramming itself and you can literally achieve anything by installing the right program at both these times. Be conscious of what you are thinking about at both these times of the day. If, before sleeping, you have thoughts of all those things that went wrong during the day, then you are programming your subconscious mind for more such wrong experiences in your life.

REPEAT, REPEAT, REPEAT

Our subconscious mind loves repetition. Repeat to yourself what you want to manifest in your life. This is called self-hypnosis. We humans can use the power of a subconscious mind to fulfill our desires and live the life we always wanted or we could use it for cribbing, complaining and making things worse for ourselves. The choice is always ours. So, use the power of repetition to imprint anything you want in life in your subconscious mind and be ready to experience the fruits of the seeds you are sowing.

There are various other techniques through which our subconscious mind could be reprogrammed and these are:

1. THE WATER TECHNIQUE.

One of the ways to reprogram our subconscious mind for what we want is through the water we drink. Now let's first understand the science behind it. **Dr. Masaru Emoto,** a famous Japanese scientist, claimed in his water experiment that "HUMAN CONSCIOUSNESS COULD AFFECT THE MOLECULAR STRUCTURE OF WATER." He did an experiment on water where he took water in different jars from the same source and exposed these jars to different words, phrases, pictures and music like "I love you," "I hate you," "You are a fool," and "You are a genius." After 24 hours when the water was frozen, it was found that the frozen crystals of the water under a microscope labeled "I hate you" and "you are a fool" were very ugly and messy, whereas the water crystals of "I love you" and "you are a genius" were very attractive and were shaped like a beautiful diamond. This experiment with water proved that **water has memory**. This was the biggest experiment that helped mankind.

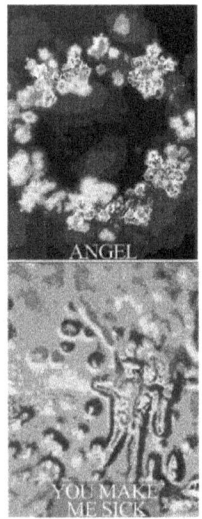
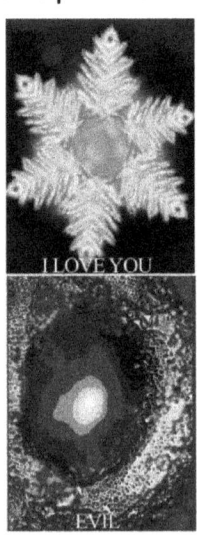
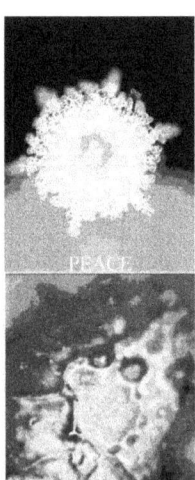
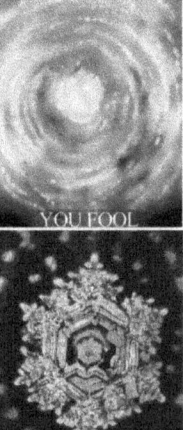

This experiment by **Dr. Masaru Emoto** proved that words could help to change the structure of molecules present in water. Now that we humans have 70-75% of water inside us, you could change your life by drinking water after affirming what you want to experience in your life or you could also write what you want on a piece of paper and stick that paper on a water bottle or jar and then after a few hours, drink that water. By doing so, you are rewiring yourself for what you want in your life. This water technique would help you reprogram your subconscious mind to achieve your dream life. Let's understand it with an example: Suppose you want more money in life, so you can write on a piece of paper, "I am a magnet to money," or "Money loves me and I love money," or "I am now earning 5 lakh rupees per month." Keep it in the present tense, as our subconscious mind works in the present. Now stick this on your water bottle or glass. As everything is energy, these words too carry their own energy, which would then be absorbed by the water. You can speak such words by visualizing what you want, holding the glass of water in both hands so that water memorizes your words and then drink this water. In this way, you are reprogramming your subconscious mind with positive words. By doing this repeatedly, you will succeed in becoming what you want to be.

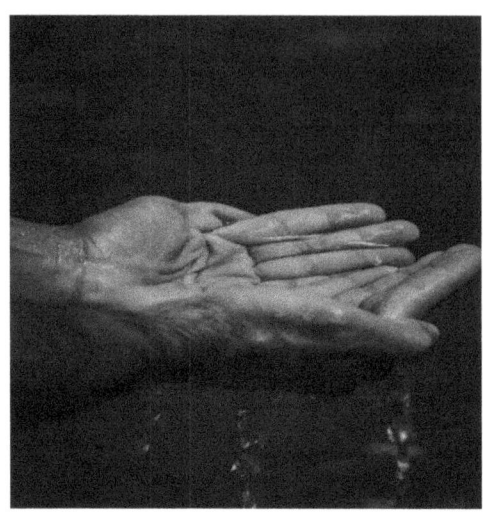

Let's connect science with our religious beliefs:

Have you ever been to a religious place? You must have been. Let me ask you: "Why in religious places do we get that water that we call "AMRIT" or "JAL" joining our hands with so much love and respect?

Don't you think it's only that water that's part of our lives? Then why do we take that Amrit with so much love and respect? It is because water has consciousness. Water has memory. When the "Shabad" or "Mantras" are chanted at religious places, that plain water absorbs those high-frequency words and thus this plain water turns into holy water and we call it "AMRIT" or "JAL.". So, use the consciousness of water to manifest what you want to achieve in your life.

2. AFFIRMATIONS:

Words are the most powerful tool to rewire your subconscious mind, as we have already learned that our subconscious mind can be reprogrammed by repetition. So, this could be done with the words we speak on a repetitive basis. Affirmations are the words and phrases that help us to change our thoughts and beliefs and gradually a new, better thought and belief is formed. When our beliefs are better and more positive, the same shows up in our lives in the form of our experiences.

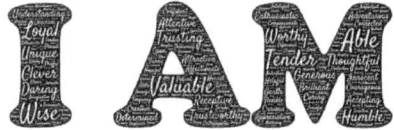

Affirmations work as auto-suggestions. Start with "I am," as "I am" is the creative power and what you say for yourself becomes your reality. Whatever you put after "I am" you become that person. Be conscious of what you put after "I am," as it shapes your reality.

This could be a good example: If you have always said, "I am good for nothing" or "I can't do anything in life," these negative statements, if repeated multiple times, would now become part of your subconscious mind and ultimately, your beliefs, your personality, your decision-making, your body language and your confidence would be exactly as the words you said and then the Laws of the Universe would put forth before you every situation, circumstance or person to prove that you are truly good for nothing. So, keep a check on the words you use. The universe is always listening. Replace "I am good for nothing" with "I am more than enough" and "I can't do it " with "I can do it this way." Start loving and respecting yourself. Love and respect who you are. Involve yourself in self-love. Never pass the mirror without complimenting yourself or giving a high five. *"Celebrate being you."* Never use any negative words or statements about yourself, such as "I am stupid," "I am not beautiful," or "I am not that smart." Know your words, as words have a deep impact on the workings of your mind and take control of your life.

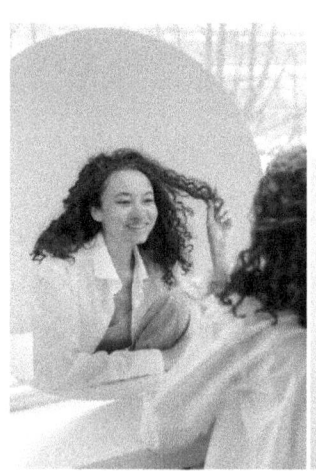
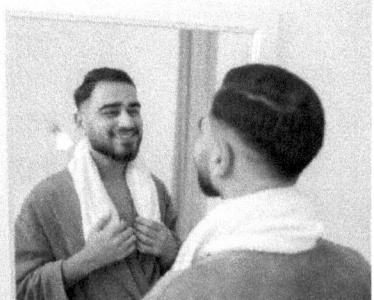

How to frame affirmations: Keep in mind the following important points while framing your affirmations:

1. Specific end result.

Don't focus on the process. Frame an affirmation that you have achieved your desired goal. Don't go into the "how" of achieving it.

2. As if it is already done.

Frame your affirmations as if they are already done. Example: I am rich, I am a celebrity and I am prosperous.

3. Add emotions.

As feelings play a major role in manifestation, you must feel what you are saying and add enough emotion to your affirmations. Example: I am loving it; I am excited; I am happy and grateful; I am surprised.

4. Create happiness before saying affirmations.

Don't say affirmations to create happiness. Instead, create happiness first and then say affirmation so that you can vibrate to that frequency. You must feel what you are saying to match that frequency and attract the same in your life.

Affirmations are repeating the words or phrases to yourself as if that thing or situation is here in this moment. It is always in the present continuous tense. It should be a positive statement, as if it were already done. Example: Let's suppose you want to be rich. Now the affirmation would be "I am rich"," I am prosperous," "I am abundant," and it's never in the future. It is always in the present moment. You must feel your affirmation to catch the frequency.

When you start affirming these positive statements slowly and slowly, they will form a part of your subconscious mind and gradually, they will be proved by the universe in your life. This is how affirmations help change our lives, and words have a deep impact on the workings of our mind.

Affirmations could help you to rewire your brain for health, wealth, success, abundance and prosperity.

Instead of saying, "I am ill," repeat, "I am healthy."

Instead of saying, "I am poor," repeat, "I am rich."

Instead of saying, "I am weak," repeat, "I am strong."

It is important to affirm positive words because what you say about yourself comes looking for you. If you say, "I am healthy," health comes looking for you. If you say, "I am wealthy," wealth comes looking for you. Whatever you want for yourself, start repeating those words or statements as affirmations daily in your mind and loudly so that you listen to those positive statements and see yourself living with that reality on the screen of your mind. Once you start realizing the power of your words, you won't just say anything.

You can use affirmations in so many ways. You can make affirmation cards, or you can use these affirmations as a password for your PC, like "Iamcreator," "Iamlove," or "Iamamazing." You can arrange your app folders and give affirmations to them. For the social media folder, you can give affirmations like "I am connected with the world." You can write affirmations on sticky notes and paste them on the refrigerator or mirror, or you can keep them hidden in different places between your clothes, drawers and notebooks. How beautiful would it be when you suddenly get these in your hands? You could be so creative with the affirmations.

You could also put on headphones and just play the affirmations of what you want in your life. It could be about health, wealth or anything you want to manifest in your life and your subconscious mind would learn this new program.

You must believe the words you say as affirmations. Feel your affirmations, as feeling is the secret. Until and unless you believe them that you deserve wealth, health, abundance and prosperity, it will not manifest in your life because you are saying it to your conscious mind, which would reject the statement saying that it is a lie. You must speak and feel the emotions of every affirmation that you practice repeatedly so that your conscious and subconscious mind get convinced by the words you are saying and sooner or later, your subconscious mind will hold that belief and do anything in its power to make it your reality.

Below is a list of a few affirmations that could help you reprogram your mind in a positive way.

1. I am reliable.
2. I am an inspiration.
3. I am trustworthy.
4. I am loved.
5. I am a positive person.
6. I am humble.
7. I am a giver.
8. I am grounded and rooted.
9. I am aligned with prosperity.
10. I am an achiever.
11. I am kind.
12. I am generous.
13. I am divinely protected.
14. I am a genius.
15. I am here to enjoy my journey.
16. I am connected with my higher consciousness.
17. I am always at the right place at the right time.
18. I am in love with who I am.
19. I am calm.

20. I am at peace.

21. I am open to receiving miracles.

22. I am getting better and better every day.

23. I am intelligent and focused.

24. I am motivated.

25. I am brilliant.

26. I am authentic.

27. I am fortunate.

28. I am beautiful.

29. I am powerful.

30. I am passionate about my life and my people.

31. I am more than enough.

32. I am creating wonderful experiences on this earth.

33. I am loving.

34. I am guided by the Supreme Power.

35. I am whole.

36. I am blessed.

37. I am now enjoying a life of abundance.

38. I am a magnet for miracles.

39. I am relaxed and peaceful.

40. I am a magnet for all the good things in my life.

3. *<u>WORDS HAVE POWER.</u>*

Words have power; never forget that. Choose your words wisely. Every word you speak has its own frequency and vibrations. They have power. Don't talk about your current reality. Speak that reality that you want to experience, as if you are experiencing it now, to get into that vibrational match of your desired life. Never say, "I don't have money." Instead, repeat, "I have more than enough money in my bank account." Whenever you speak and think anything negative, immediately use the words "CANCEL, CANCEL, CANCEL" or "CUT, CUT, CUT" as every word has its own frequency and so these words too have the frequency to cancel your negative thoughts and words you speak to manifest.

Whenever you have any complaints about anything or anyone around you, instantly start focusing on what you want rather than what you don't want. Let's say if you have a complaint that your husband or partner is too angry, immediately shift your focus to "My partner or husband is calm and peaceful always."

Many times, we feel that things are not working in our favor. Whenever I feel that things are not going my way, I repeat the empowering words I learned from Louise Hay, which say,

"All is well. Everything is always working out for my highest good. Out of this situation, only good will come. I am safe and protected."

This instantly gives me a positive attitude and makes me feel relaxed and calm. You too can practice these.

Whatever you think about, whatever you talk about, whatever you focus on, is exactly what is going to happen to you in your life. Whenever you have a conversation with someone, ask yourself these questions often:

What am I talking about? Do I want to experience it in my life?

What am I listening to? Do I want to experience it in my life?

Your answers to the above questions will tell you what you need to do next. If you hear others complaining about something, withdraw your attention; don't get involved in their battle. And if they share something exciting, give them your full attention and feel that joy as if it's your own experience of life.

Talk more about what you love. It could be anything-the luxurious cars you love, the beautiful home you love to live in, your loving relationship with your partner, your love for travelling-talk as much as you can about the things you love the most and get yourself to the frequency and vibrations of those things and see the magic happening in your life.

4. *WHAT WE SEE IS WHAT WE ATTRACT.*

As our subconscious mind thinks in images, it is important to keep a check on what we see. In today's digital world, we are all exposed to so much information that most of us are in the habit of watching anything, even the worst of incidents, on repeated mode. Do you know that these images are going deep in your mind? For the happy and prosperous life, you want, what type of images should you hold in your mind? The day I learned this, I became very conscious of what I was watching, as everything gets downloaded into our subconscious mind. Good things happen to those who have good thoughts. You must have heard "Garbage in, Garbage out."

Many are in the habit of starting the day by reading newspapers or watching news, which gives 90% of negative news to your mind early in the morning. Now, what do you think your day would be like? Many are in the habit of checking out social media on their phones first thing in the morning. By checking out our social media apps most of the time we fill our minds with all the crap and unhealthy images and then we start our day and we expect our lives to be happy, fulfilled and prosperous. *Learn to unlearn what is not serving you.*

So, if you are not getting what you want, you first must unlearn and leave your old self to be a "New You."

Songs you listen to:

The songs you listen to are also recorded in your subconscious mind. Music with lyrics turns out to be subliminal messages that go straight into our subconscious mind. The lyrics of the song you listen to are recorded in your subconscious mind and would gradually turn out to be your experience of life. Choose wisely what you listen to. Check out the lyrics of the song. Question yourself, "Would I like to live it as my experience in life?" If the answer is "YES," you can listen to the song repeatedly. You can also choose to listen to affirmation songs on YouTube. Below are few songs I usually listen to.

"Money is coming to me." – Eddie Watkins Jr.

"Abundance is coming to me, right now." – Bob Baker.

"I don't chase, I attract."– Monita.

"I am "me," and that's my superpower." – Fearless soul.

"Love you zindagi." – Dear Zindagi.

"I am the best." – Phir bhi dil hai hindustani.

"I make my money stack to the roof." – Able Heart.

"I am worthy. Yes, I am." – Coax marie.

"I am my own hero" – Fearless Soul.

The list goes unending. You can add to your playlist an unlimited number of songs. Just make sure it doesn't say anything that you don't want to experience in your life, as lyrics mean affirmations and music means sound frequency. Choose consciously what you feed your mind with, as that is exactly what will show up in your life.

Gratitude is the Key

"Develop an attitude of Gratitude and give thanks for everything that happens to you"

-Brian Tracy
(An Author and Speaker)

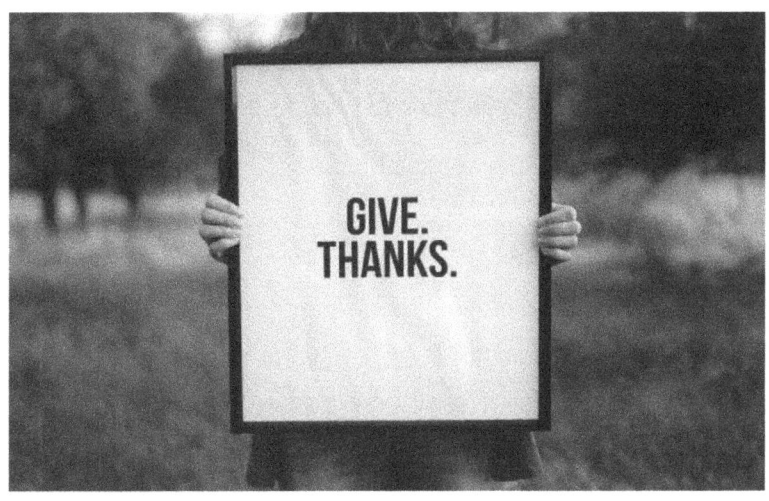

The word gratitude is derived from the Latin word "Gratus" which means "pleasing" or "thankful." Gratitude is the state of being thankful for all you have in your life.

After understanding the law of vibration, practicing "gratitude" is no longer a secret. Gratitude means being grateful. Being grateful for what the universe or God has blessed you with is the key to unlocking the doors of happiness, abundance and success in your life. To experience the richness of life, be thankful to "God," the "Universe," or you can call "Divine." You don't need to be rich, successful or happier first; rather, you have to be grateful first for what the universe has blessed you with to experience the richness of life. It is rightly said, "If you want to find happiness, find gratitude."

Now, many of you would have a long, unending list of things you don't have in your life and your next question might be, "How can I be grateful?"

Then my question to you would be:

Do you have eyes? Many people on this planet can't see, but you are blessed to see this beautiful world. You are blessed to see your loved ones. You are blessed to live your life while witnessing the beauty around you. Be grateful for these eyes.

Do you have arms and legs? Many in this world are not so blessed. Many can't walk properly. Many don't have arms. Be grateful that you are living with your arms and legs and doing whatever you want to.

And even before these, the major reason to be grateful for:

Do you have an index finger? Of course, you do. Put it under your nose. Could you sense air moving in and out of your nose? Be grateful that "YOU ARE ALIVE" and when you are alive, anything could be possible. Many have left the world today. Be grateful that you are not one of them. Celebrate each day of your life because you are alive.

If you have food to eat, clothes to wear and shelter over your head, then be grateful. Be thankful. "YOU ARE BLESSED." However, we humans are actually programmed to complain. Ever since childhood, we have watched others complain about the success of other people. Mr. X has so much money- luxury cars, a bungalow but I don't have that. Remember, the laws of the universe are always working. When you feel grateful for the experiences, things and people in your life, the whole universe supports you and blesses you with more of the good experiences, things, and people around you. Start saying "thank you" for your job that helps you feed your family, pay for your kids' education and live your life. Although it is not your dream job, the money you receive from this job helps you in many ways. So, be grateful. Many are unemployed. Imagine losing your job. How would your life be? Imagine not having food on your table. Imagine not having clean water to drink. Would your life be as comfortable as it is now? Imagine your life without your loved ones. How would your life be then?

Be grateful for all the things you have in your life, and don't take them for granted. Practicing gratitude would reprogram your mind to find the good around you. It's the key to your happier, prosperous, abundant, and rich version.

If you saw the seed of always being grateful in your mind and always counting your blessings, life would become much easier and happier.

Say "thank you" to your body. It's making a great effort to keep you alive. Your heart is pumping. Your kidneys and lungs are working for you. Your brain is functioning. Your whole body is working to keep you alive. It's doing a great job. Don't forget to say "thank you" to it.

Say "thank you" to everyone you meet for everything they did for you. Say "thank you" when you enter your home. Say "thank you" when you switch on your PC. Say "thank you" on your way home, looking around at the beautiful things that nature has blessed us with. Say "thank you" for everything and for everyone in your life.

Complaining about people, things, and situations would never serve you. Get rid of your complaints.

> *"Gratitude is a law of increase and complaint is a law of decrease."*
>
> **-Florence Scovel Shinn**
> **(An American artist)**

As everything is "energy," the vibrations you give out to the universe when you are grateful for everything around you come back to you with more great things to be grateful for. We all spend too much energy on what others have instead of being grateful for what we have. Gratitude helps shift your focus from lack to abundance. Giving gratitude is the most common technique followed by all successful people in the world. They give thanks for all they have and this makes them focus on the positive aspects of their lives and they become the attraction point for all the better and more positive things in life.

"Most people are grateful after they receive good, but to make all your wishes come true and change your entire life by filling it with riches in every area, you must be grateful before and after."

THE MAGIC
(A book by Rhonda Byrne)

VARIOUS TECHNIQUES TO PRACTICE GRATITUDE:

Here are some techniques that I learned on my journey of personal development.You could practice different techniques in a month or you could try one technique for one month and shift to another to enjoy it in different ways. The only purpose is to keep yourself focused on the good, keep your vibrations high and make gratitude a part of your life.

1. Take a journal and name it *"Gratitude Journal."* Now, every day, write 10 random things you are grateful for. It could be your family, your home, your bed, AC, computer, air, water, food, your body, health, beauty, skin, hair, eyes, the air you breathe- anything that you are blessed with. You could also express gratitude for those things that you want to manifest in your life by feeling the emotions of already receiving them in the present moment.

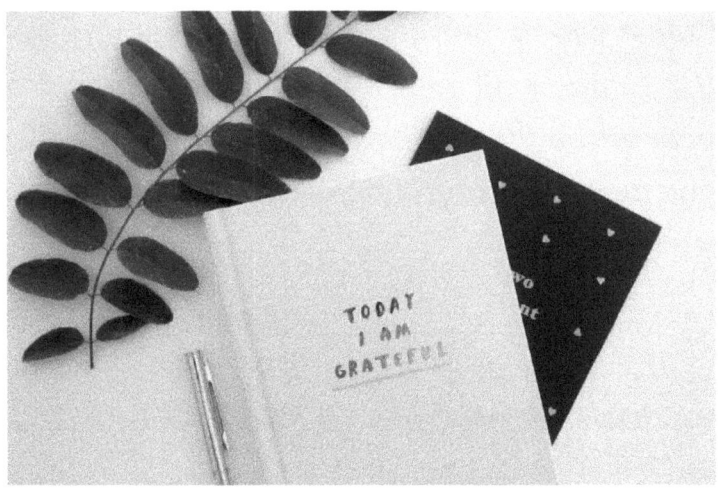

2. The other way to practice gratitude is to do 15 minutes of *"Gratitude Walk"* every day in nature. Let the universe know how grateful you are for everything that the universe has blessed you with.

3. There is one more way to practice gratitude. It could be easily done with your kids, too. Take a jar, decorate it beautifully and name it *"Gratitude Jar."* Now each day, take a slip and write 5-10 things you are grateful for and put them in the jar. After one month, you will be surprised to see how blessed you are.

4. Another way to express gratitude is to write **"A Gratitude Letter to the Universe,"** thanking the universe for all it has blessed you with. Start with:

Dear Universe,

"I am so happy and grateful that you blessed me with......................." (Continue what you are blessed with and what you want to manifest in your life, giving gratitude in advance as if it has already manifested in your life.)

5. ***Go seven days without complaining.*** Try this out for a week. For 7 days, don't complain about anything in your life. Anything means anything. There are no excuses for that. Just for a week, say "thank you" to everyone you meet and to everything you have. No matter how difficult the situation is, just focus on being thankful for the lesson it has come to teach you. You will see how easily you can heal the problem and raise your vibrations. And if, out of your old complaining pattern, a negative thought comes into your mind, you can remind yourself, "I am going to say what I want to experience or manifest in my life."

6. The other way of shifting your focus from lack to abundance could be that whenever you feel negative for someone, ***"snap your fingers"(Chutki bajao)*** change the thought pattern and say "Thank you" for the lessons you learned. Just with a snap of your fingers, shift your focus on the positives of that person. This would allow you to instantly shift your vibes from feeling negative to feeling positive about another person or situation.

7. **Finding your Gratitude Rock**- You can take any rock that attracts you, name it "Gratitude Rock," and keep that rock in your pocket every day with you wherever you go. Whenever you touch that rock, think of one thing you are grateful for and every night before sleeping, you can hold that rock and say "thank you" for the best things that happened during the day. This would keep your focus on the good that happened to you rather than cribbing for the things that went wrong throughout the day.

8. Another way to practice gratitude in today's digital world could be by dropping a *"thank you message"* to someone and sharing how that person has made your life better.

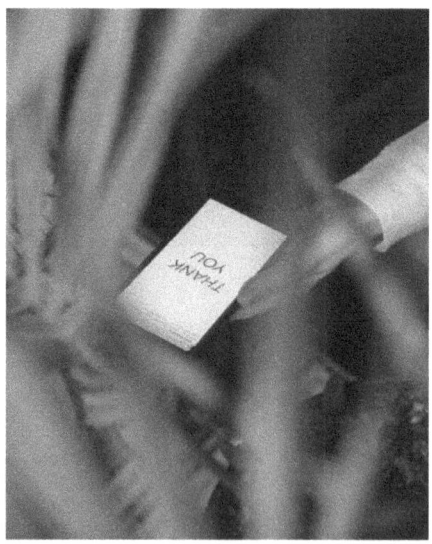

9. **Sending some flowers or gifts along with a thank-you letter**. You could go a step ahead and send

flowers, a small gift with a thank-you note, or a letter explaining how the person has influenced your life and that you are grateful for all that person has done for you.I have done this personally, and the happiness and joy I experienced when the person was surprised is just phenomenal. You just start vibing so high.

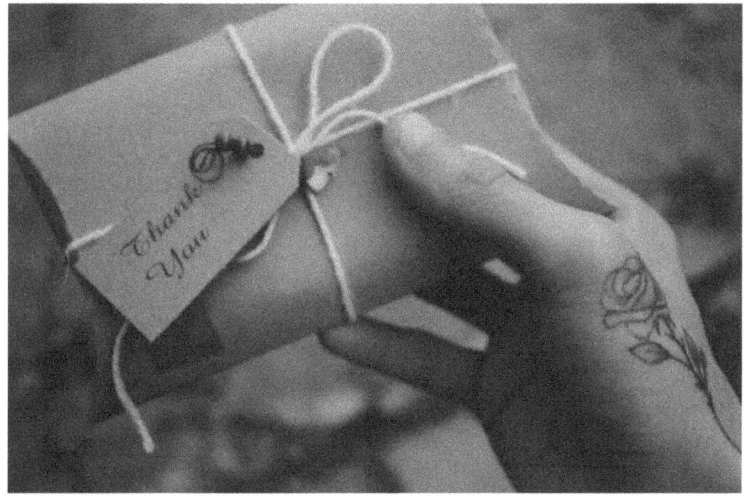

So stop complaining, criticizing and crying, and start being thankful for all you have to attract more of what you want in your life. Start appreciating the people around you. Say "thank you" to them often. Let them know that you are grateful for their acts of kindness, support, and love for you. Appreciate the little things around you.

GRATITUDE LIST

Below is the gratitude list. This list would give you an idea of the things and experiences you could be grateful for.

1. Universe/God/Divine.
2. Life.
3. Family.
4. Health.
5. Money.
6. Food.
7. Home.
8. Job.
9. Clean water to drink.
10. Education.
11. Teachers.
12. Wisdom.
13. Knowledge.
14. Weekends with family.
15. Pets.
16. Friends.
17. Relatives.
18. Holidays.
19. Trips.

20. Parents.

21. Comforts.

22. Favorite memories.

23. Bed for sound sleep.

24. Air Conditioner.

25. Refrigerator

26. Mobile.

27. Vehicles.

28. Garden.

29. Flowers.

30. Birds and animals.

31. Experiences.

32. Struggles.

33. Life lessons you learned.

34. Children.

35. Spouse.

36. Skin.

37. Hair.

38. Body.

39. Wisdom.

40. Physical and mental health.

You could also be grateful for this book in your hands, for this new knowledge that came your way and could give a new direction to your life.

And the list goes on. Be grateful for every little and big thing and all the experiences in your life, as everything contributes to making you reach this moment of your life.

"Whatever you appreciate and give thanks for will increase in your life."

Sanaya Roman
(A Spiritual teacher and an author)

The 2 ways to Elevated Emotions

Now, after learning all about energy, the laws of the Universe and the powers of our mind, let's find out the two most common ways to experience elevated emotions each day. Elevated emotions are emotions of high vibrations like peace, relaxation, joy and happiness. The two easiest ways to experience them are through meditation and dancing. They both help in changing your energy and making you feel those high vibes.

MEDITATION

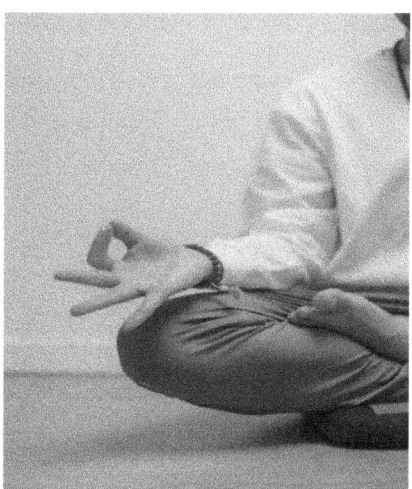

Meditation raises our vibrations. It is one of the techniques that helps in the manifestation process too. Every day, find some time and sit in complete silence with yourself. Go deep inside and listen to what your heart says. Find your inner voice, and you will find peace and guidance for your life. Meditation produces oxytocin in your body and the more you produce oxytocin, the more it will give you the emotions of love, fulfillment, compassion and forgiveness.

It is a way of getting connected with our inner being. Meditation could be done with various meditative music too. However, I usually practice meditation just by sitting in silence to connect with my inner being or higher consciousness, starting with inhaling and exhaling. I sit in silence for about 15-20 minutes to hear what my inner being or higher consciousness has to communicate to me and I must say there have been awakening moments for me. I usually get answers to all my questions during meditation.

Meditation is just like a GPS system. As the GPS system tells us which route we have to follow to reach our destination, in the same way meditation is connecting with our inner being, our inner guidance that knows all the way to our dream life.

Do you know that we are all here for some purpose? Until and unless you could find your purpose on this planet, only then would you be able to feel contentment with your life and to understand your purpose start connecting more with your inner guidance, your inner being, as it has all the answers. No one on this earth knows what your purpose is for being on this planet. It's only your inner guidance, your inner being, that knows it all. So, never ask anyone else about your existence, your purpose, your dreams or the route to follow for your dreams. All these answers are within you. All you have to do is build a connection with yourself. Your inner being will guide you from time to time through impulses.

"I received a strong impulse to start writing something and slowly and gradually, it turned out to be a book in your hands."

Your inner guidance speaks to you through impulses. Whatever impulse you have, never try to question it. Rather, start acting on your impulses from that very moment. Never ask anyone for their opinion on your impulses. They would never understand your story. Just start by taking action on your impulses. It couldn't be wrong. It's always right. Do exactly what you get an impulse for. Listen to your inner guidance always. Learn to surrender to your inner guidance, the universe and the God within you. Never doubt or question your inner guidance, as it knows your journey and your purpose for being on this planet.

DANCING

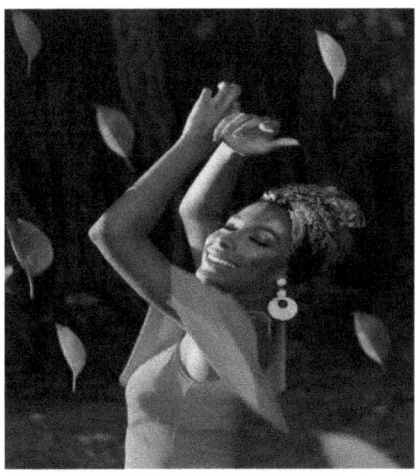

Dancing is one of the ways to make yourself vibrate high. Dancing is an expression of happiness, joy and fulfillment. During dance, our brain releases 1400 happy hormones. Make your brain used to oxytocin and dopamine. These are happy hormones. By doing dancing and meditation for 30 consecutive days, your mind will become addicted to these happy hormones and it will find reasons to be happy and joyful even in your biggest worries. Get your mind and body used to happy hormones by dancing, meditating or doing whatever makes you feel happy. You are rewiring your mind for happiness and joy instead of complaining, cribbing and crying. Most of us have become used to stress hormones and our brain finds unnecessary reasons to complain and cry, sometimes even over minor things.

Dancing helps make you feel those high vibrations of love, joy and happiness. When we dance, we are in a happy and joyful mood and the laws of the universe say that what energy you give, you get back. So, you become a magnet to attract people situations and events of more joy and happiness in your life. Dance for 15 to 20 minutes each day, choosing the song with the right lyrics to communicate the same message to the universe and to attract it into your reality.

Script your life

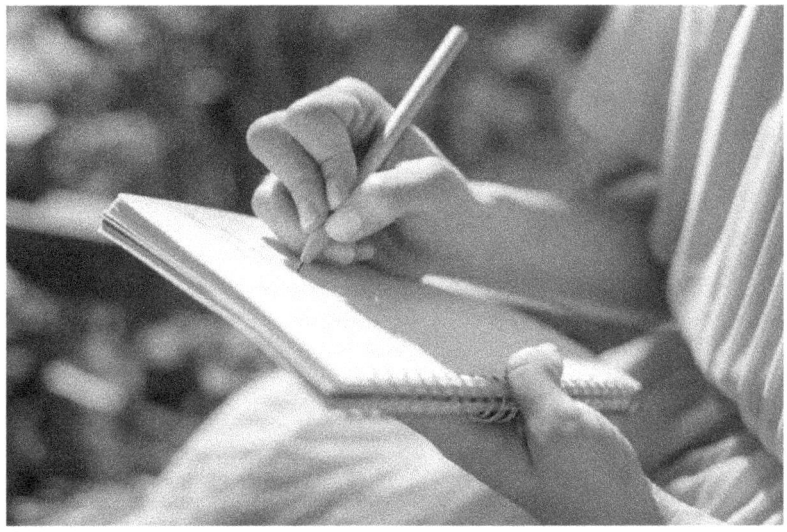

"Script your life." Yes, you read it right. You can literally write down on paper what you want in your life and how you would feel if it were already done. Scripting is another way of manifesting what you want in life. Scripting is a very powerful way of manifesting your desires. Every important contract or deal is always done on paper. Everything important is always done in writing. It is said, "If it's not on paper, it's vapor." Write down the list of things you want to attract into your life. Pen down your dream as if it has already happened. It is like speaking things into existence. Scripting involves writing down your emotions, feelings and thoughts and imagining the moment when you have achieved what you want. By doing so, you get aligned with the vibrations of your goal being achieved. This again results in matching the frequency of your desires being fulfilled. The more you do it, the more you are rewiring your brain for success.

There are a few points you need to keep in mind while scripting.

1. Use the present tense as if what you want has already happened.

2. Write down how it feels to you and your emotions once it has happened in your life. Use more high-vibrational words like excited, joy, happiness, love and contentment, as high vibrations are what we need.

3. Express gratitude that it has happened in your life.

4. Put your signatures at the end with the current date.

5. Let it go.

SCRIPTING FOR MANIFESTING YOUR" DREAM HOME."

Suppose your desire is to have a "dream home." Now in scripting, you would write down, "I am so happy and grateful that I am living in my dream home. It's exactly what I wanted. It has a swimming pool and a garden, which I always wanted in my home. My garden has beautiful trees and flowers and I love the chirping of birds on my trees. My daughter enjoys swimming in her personal swimming pool now. I am so happy and grateful to the universe for blessing me with this beautiful home. Thank you, thank you, thank you, universe, for my sweet new home." The above is just a brief example of it. Add as many details as possible because the more details you add, the more clear the picture you will have in your mind. The clearer it is, the easier it is to manifest in your life.

In short, imagine a scene of your wish fulfillment and you are now sharing it with your best friend or a loved one. Feel the feelings of it being manifested, as feeling is the secret.

SCRIPTING FOR MANIFESTING YOUR "PARTNER/SPOUSE."

Let's say you want to manifest a specific person in your life, maybe your partner or spouse. Write as if he or she is already in your life. Write down what qualities he or she has. How does he or she look? What is his or her way of dressing? How does he or she talk? Which are the places you visit often together? Write down the conversations you both have. How do you feel about spending time with that person?

Write everything in the present tense as if you have already met that person and you both are in a relationship. Get into the vibrations of that person already existing in your life and manifest your dream partner.

IN THE SAME WAY, YOU CAN SCRIPT FOR ANYTHING YOU WANT TO MANIFEST IN YOUR LIFE. THE ONLY RULE YOU NEED TO FOLLOW IS THAT YOUR DESIRE IS FULFILLED. NOW PEN DOWN YOUR THOUGHTS AND FEELINGS OF YOUR DESIRE FULFILLED IN THE PRESENT MOMENT.

THINGS YOU WANT TO ATTRACT.

Make a list of things you want to attract. You can write anything you want to attract in your life. Below are a few examples:

1. I attract love and laughter into my life.
2. I attract money into my life.
3. I attract luxurious lifestyle.
4. I attract being an author.
5. I attract celebrations in my life.
6. I attract my dream home.
7. I attract my dream car.
8. I attract loving, kind and supportive people into my life.
9. I attract health and wealth into my life.
10. I attract success, abundance and prosperity into my life.

WHAT ALL YOU LOVE.

Make a list of 50-100 things you would love to enjoy in your life. Below is a list of 10 things to help you know what it would be like.

1. I love luxuries.

2. I love peace.
3. I love mansions.
4. I love nature.
5. I love money.
6. I love abundance.
7. I love prosperity.
8. I love name and fame.
9. I love awards.
10. I love happiness.

When you prepare the list of 100 things that you love to enjoy in your life, you have tuned yourself to the vibrations and the frequency of those things. It doesn't need any explanation about how we feel when we think about the things we love. We all feel happy and joyful.

DECLARATION FOR THE MONTH.

You could also write down the "Declaration for the Month." It is done on the first of every month to declare how your month will be. A declaration declares in advance how you want your month would be. In a declaration, you write down all the things and experiences that you want to manifest in an upcoming month.

It starts like, "Thank you, Universe, for the great and amazing beginnings this month. This month is going to be a month full of love, laughter, luxuries, abundance, prosperity and lots and lots of wonderful experiences. Thank you, Universe, for incredible guidance and unfoldings this month

(Continue with what you want to manifest and experience in the upcoming month.)

End up your declaration with Thank you, Thank you, Thank you, written three times with your signatures and current date on it.

In this way, you take hold of your powers to manifest what you want to experience in your life and through scripting, you let the universe and your subconscious mind know what you want from your life.

Visualization

"Visualization is where everything starts."

-Bob Proctor
(Canadian Author and a Life Coach)

Visualization is the most powerful technique to bring your dreams to reality. We have already discussed that our subconscious mind thinks in images and does not differentiate between imagination and reality. So sit down for 10 to 15 minutes each day, closing your eyes and imagining the images of you winning that award you always wanted, your dream home you want to live in, getting married to your dream partner, achieving your goals, or anything else you want to manifest. Bring those scenes before your eyes. Get it very clear. Try to get as detailed and clear as you possibly can. Imagine every detail around you. Feel the emotion of this event happening in your life right now. Feel the emotions of it through your senses. Use your five senses. Make it as real as you possibly can. The more real it seems to you during visualization, the faster it will manifest in your life. Your body does not feel the difference between an event actually taking place or you imagining it. Make your body experience right now what it feels like to live your dream moment. By doing this, you would be emitting a strong signal, a vibration of that experience taking place in your life right now and by doing this continuously, you are summoning the same event to happen in your life through the laws of the universe, which are precise and clear. Do it daily. The more you feel it, the more you are attracting what you want into your life. Visualization gives your brain a target to achieve anything that you want. Your subconscious mind only works in the present. You have to imagine that you have it now. It can't reason.

PROCESS OF VISUALIZATION

Do this process for 15-20 minutes once or twice a day, consistently and experience the magic of visualization.

1. Decide what you want. It could be your dream car, your dream home, your desired job, an award, or any experience you want to manifest in your life.
2. Believe you can have it; you deserve it and it's possible for you.
3. Close your eyes and visualize having what you want as if you already have it.
4. Feel the feeling of having it now.
5. Focus on being grateful for all you have.
6. Release it to the universe. Let it go.
7. Trust the universe to manifest it.
8. Don't question "how." The universe has unlimited ways to make things happen and we call them miracles.

Don't go into how it's going to manifest in your life. This universe has unlimited ways to manifest anything we desire in our lives. Don't fall into the trap of logical thinking, as our universe works in miraculous ways beyond our imagination to bring forth what we are aligned with. "How" your desire would be fulfilled is none of your concern. The power of your subconscious mind and the laws of the universe will bring you what you want. The "how" is not for you to think about. Your only work is to feel the emotions of your desires fulfilled in the present moment. And let the magic of divine forces reveal to you how it could become your reality.

"If you do just a little research, it is going to become evident to you that anyone who has ever accomplished anything did not know how they were going to do it. They only knew they were going to do it."

- Bob Proctor
(Canadian Author and Life Coach)

We all use the power of imagination and visualization, consciously or unconsciously. Most of us use these powers against ourselves. We usually think about what could go wrong, imagining the worst of circumstances for ourselves. Instead, use your mental faculties in your favor. I remember the words I once read, which say:

"Losers visualize the penalties of failure, Winners visualize the rewards of success."

William S.Gilbert
(An English Dramatist, Poet, Illustrator and Librettist)

Don't use your imagination destructively; rather, use your imagination constructively. Use the power of visualization and imagination to think and feel the best of what could happen to you and how beautiful life could turn out to be.

Your imagination is your greatest creative power. Everything that you enjoy in your life, be it your microwave, pen, computer, phone or laptop- every small and big thing-existed first in the imagination of a man and then took a physical form in your reality. It's impossible for you to have something in your life until and unless you create that picture in your mind. So, the role your imagination and visualization play in framing your life is beyond words.

Napoleon Hill too says, "Everything is first constructed in the human mind and then in the physical world." When the Wright Brothers invented an airplane, it was first the thought of imagining something that could make us fly high in the sky. Had they not imagined, an airplane would have never been in the physical world. Every invention is first created in our mind and then in the physical world.

SPEC METHOD

Helene Hadsell was an American lady known as the "Contest Queen." She participated in almost 5,000 contests and in almost all the contests, she won something like cash, home appliances, travel and much more. She won every prize she desired, which also included a fully furnished home. When asked how she manifests everything, she shared a four-step method known as SPEC. It means

1. Select it.
2. Project it.
3. Expect it.
4. Collect it.

1. **Select it**- You choose what you want, whether it's a dream home, a car, a partner, money, winning the lottery, or a contest-whatever you desire to manifest in your life.

2. **Project it**- It's the most important one. You visualize yourself as living that desired reality. If you selected your dream home to manifest, imagine yourself living in that home and what that home would look like. Feel the vibrations and the emotions of living in your dream home "now."

3. **Expect it**-You have to live with the end result, as it has already been there in the moment.

4. **Collect it**-It's manifested.

You must believe that you have it now in the present moment, experience the feelings and emotions of living your dream at this moment and watch the universe shift in your favor every reality to make your dream come true.

Bob Proctor, a famous Canadian author and speaker, says, **"By visualizing your goal already completed, you flip your mind onto the frequency that contains the way that it will be attracted to you."**

Another study was done at the University of Chicago, where they took three groups of people and made them practice free throws.

Group A was to practice each day.

Group B was not allowed to practice at all.

Group C was allowed to practice only in their minds without touching the ball or being on the court, successfully throwing free throws for an hour a day. These groups were then followed up 30 days later and measured.

Group A was back on the court and improved by 24%.

Group B didn't show any results as they didn't practice at all.

Group C has just practiced in their minds and improved by 23%.

Just 1% less than the people that were put on the court. This shows the power of visualization.

Visualization is thus the strongest key to manifest anything you want in your life.

Now start using the powers of your mental faculties and see your life transform before your eyes.

> *"Visualization is the key to creating the reality you desire."*
>
> ***Oprah Winfrey***
> *(An American producer, actress and an Author)*

Vision Boards

"If I can see it and believe it, then I can achieve it"
And you can too.

-Arnold Schwarzenegger
(a former Governor of California
and an actor, Filmmaker, politician)

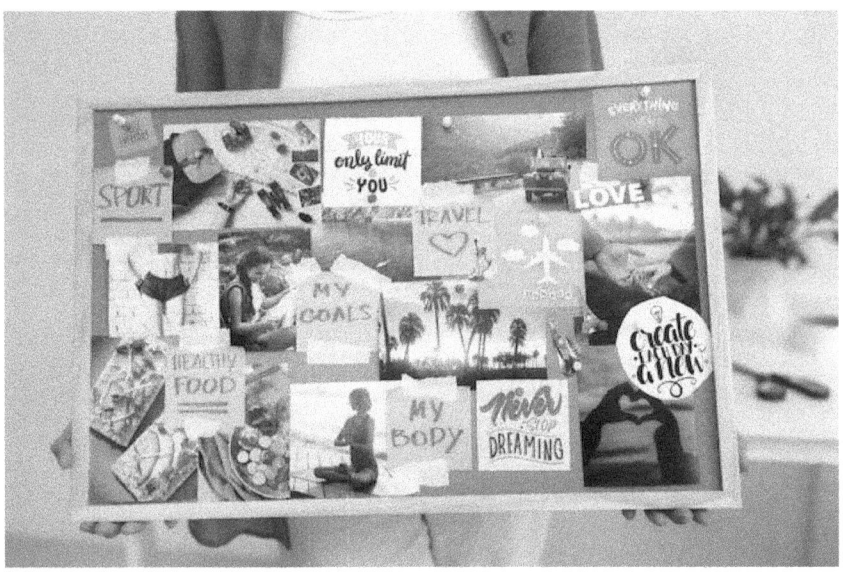

Using the vision boards is one of the techniques to rewire our subconscious mind. Vision boards play an important role in reprogramming our subconscious mind. It's about creating a board where you keep before yourself your vision of the next

6 months or 1 year that you want to achieve and experience as your reality in life. On your vision board, you can use affirmations, images, photographs, or quotes that help you visualize what you want to achieve. By preparing a vision board, you give command to your subconscious mind to know what exactly you want to achieve in your life in the upcoming months or year. Vision boards are the easiest way to rewire our subconscious mind for what we want to achieve in our lives. We humans can retain a visual image more clearly and for a longer period of time. So, making a vision board helps us to see our goals clearly, giving a clear image to our mind and therefore actualizing them in our reality.

METHOD TO MAKE A VISION BOARD.

There is a method to prepare a vision board. First, you must write down your clear goals and intentions for your future in your goal diary. It could be for the next 6 months or 1 year, like buying a home, a car, traveling to your dream destination, achieving any award, or anything else that you want. Now what you must do is find out the exact pictures that are aligned with your dream home, dream car, or the country you want to travel to. Google them. Select the images that excite you. Once you have the pictures of your dream home, car or award you always wanted, you can "Photoshop" yourself and fix your pictures with your dream. Suppose it's the picture of a dream home. You can Photoshop yourself along with your family with that home, or you can put your photo with your dream car, or you can make your award-winning photos with the help of Photoshop. Now you must paste these on a piece of cardboard or a chart. You can paste all the photos of your vision that you want to manifest. Now write affirmations below those pictures. Let's say you have a photo of your dream car, you can write below this photo, "I am now driving my brand-new car." If you have a photo of yourself with your dream home, the affirmation below could be, "I am now living in my dream home happily." If you have an award-winning picture of yours, you can write, "I have won the award (name of the award you intend to win)."

You can also create a digital vision board on your phone or computer as your wallpaper by making a collage of all the photos that you select.

WHAT DOES "VISION BOARD" DO?

Now the question would be, "What does the vision board do?" A vision board helps create a strong and powerful image in your mind of what you actually want to achieve. Therefore, it keeps you focused, motivated and accountable, which helps you achieve what you want. It helps you visualize your goals. It gives a success image to your mind. By looking at it every day, you immerse yourself in a visual image of what you want to achieve. It then creates a positive and powerful image of your goal in your mind.

As we have already learned, our subconscious mind thinks in images and to rewire our subconscious mind, the most important time of the day is the time when we wake up and 5 minutes before we go to sleep. So, place this vision board in front of your bed and see it as the first thing in the morning and the last thing before you go to sleep at night. Now what happens is that our subconscious mind does not know the difference between imagination and reality. If these images were seen regularly at both times, they would get imprinted in your subconscious mind and your subconscious mind would take them as your new reality. When we do it on a consistent basis, these get imprinted in our subconscious mind and sooner or later, they will become our reality.

WHY MAKE A VISION BOARD?

A vision board constantly reminds you about your goals and visions for a particular time. It gives you a clear idea of how much you have to achieve and what actions you need to take to reach those goals.

The key areas to consider and make goals about on vision boards are:

1. Start with expressing gratitude: Start with the words "Thank you Universe" on your vision board to come true "in advance."

2. Financial Goals: Write down your financial goals. What exactly would you like to achieve in terms of your financial goals in the next 12 months? Collect the images that align with your goals and inspire you to work for them.

3. Family and Relationship Goals: Write down how you want your family and relationships to flourish in the

next 12 months and find the exact pictures that are aligned with your vision.

4. Health and Wellness Goals: How do you see yourself in the area of your health in the next 12 months? It could be a goal of reducing all that excess weight, eating a healthy diet, or starting with yoga or meditation. Collect the exact pictures that inspire you to achieve your goals.

5. Travel Goals: Collect images of the places you want to travel to in the next 12 months. It could be a national or international trip. It could be with family or on solo trips.

6. Knowledge Goals: What is something new you would like to learn in the next 6 to 12 months? Think over it. It could be taking some seminars with your favorite speaker or coaches. It could be reading a certain number of books by the time the year ends. It could be learning the AI tools.

Collect the images and place them on your vision board to keep your conscious and subconscious minds focused on what exactly you have to achieve in the upcoming year and to take actions accordingly.

Richness of Health

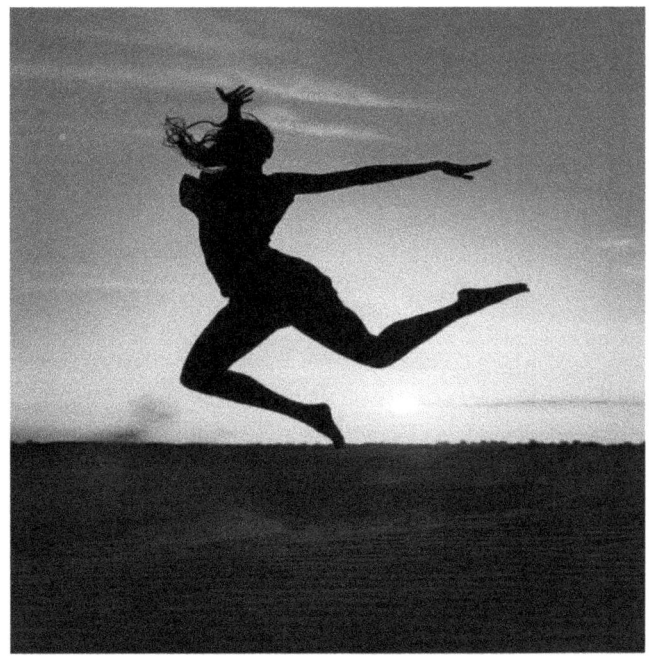

It is now scientifically proven that our health is totally dependent on our thoughts, emotions and mental patterns. Our physical health is directly related to the thoughts we have and the emotions we feel, as our mind and body are interconnected and our thoughts influence our physical health.

Therefore, learn to examine your thoughts. Do you often think of good health? or Do you often listen to the diseases or health issues of others? Are you the one who is interested in sharing information about diseases or health issues? Are you the one who is always stressed or tensed? If you are the one who hears a lot about diseases and focuses your energy on learning more about the symptoms of different diseases, you will end up manifesting those in your life. Instead, give your energy and attention to perfect health. Ask yourself often, "How would it feel if I were enjoying a fit and healthy body?" "How would it feel to be relaxed, calm and peaceful all the time?" How would it feel if I always felt energetic? Think and feel the emotions of you enjoying that fit and healthy body. The illness is always the body's way of telling you that you are on the wrong track and that you need to change. Just look for what needs to be released without complaining. Your body is a mirror of your thoughts and feelings and is always listening to you. It is scientifically proven now that all diseases are self-created. You attract health issues just because of your own limiting beliefs. You create a mental atmosphere for a disease to be created. The universe totally supports your inner dialogue and your experiences are the outcomes of your inner dialogue only. If you hold the emotions of resentment, guilt, fear or criticism for others, it creates several health issues.

Your body is a mirror of your inner thoughts and is always communicating with you in a variety of ways.

Your illness is a reminder to change something that is not right. It's giving you the opportunity to change your thoughts. We often forget to admire our bodies and what they do. We usually look into our bodies when we feel pain or discomfort. Start giving unconditional love to your body. Stand in front of the mirror and give love to each body part.

WRITING A LOVE LETTER TO YOUR BODY.

Write a love letter to your body. Thank your body and each body part for performing their functions properly. Thank your heart, kidneys, lungs, eyes, ears, hair, arms, legs, pancreas, digestive system and other organs for working to keep you alive and making you experience this beautiful journey called "life." Be kind to yourself, as your physical health is just a projection of your mental health. Use positive phrases for your health. Take care of your health. Give some time to physical activity and indulge in eating healthy food. Work on your beliefs to manifest good health. Give love to yourself. Show some love to your body.

We all deserve good health. It's our birth right. Check your beliefs about your health. If you believe that after a certain age you will contract diseases, you are then likely to get one, as this is your belief.

Repeat "I am free from my illness now," "I am getting healthier with each passing day," "I enjoy perfect health now," "I am free from all the pains and sufferings in my body," and "I am fine, healthy and happy."

Visualize yourself in a healthy, happy state. See yourself doing everything you want to do. Whenever the thought of illness comes to your mind, repeat "cancel" three times, as this will nullify your negative thought and then repeat the positive affirmation about your health. Become deaf to anything negative about health. You must be deaf to all the negative statements like, "health deteriorates with age," "illness is a way of living," and "health, once gone, can't be restored." Free yourself from such limiting beliefs about health.

Always focus on what you want rather than what you don't want.

When you look in the mirror, look straight into your eyes and give love to each body part every single day. For any disease, pain or illness in your body, repeat, "I am willing to release the pattern in me that has created this disease or illness."

Think about perfect health. Visualize yourself celebrating your 100th birthday to give your mind a mental picture of you living more than 100 years and that too in a healthy state. Don't talk about your ill health with others, even when you could feel that illness, as by talking and speaking about your illness, you are affirming more of it. Instead, repeat, "I am well; I am fine." The more you repeat it, the more you are *giving command to your mind to keep the body fit, as there is undoubtedly a mind- body connection.*

VISUALIZATION TECHNIQUE FOR HEALTH.

Start visualizing and thinking about yourself with perfect health and a perfect body and try to ignite those emotions in you with perfect physical and mental health. See yourself competing with the young ones. See everyone admiring you for your fit and healthy body. See yourself thanking your body for being fit and active. Get yourself aligned with the idea of being healthy, active and energetic all the time.

HO'OPONOPONO PRAYER FOR HEALTH.

Practice this prayer for your body and health. Completely release all the negative emotions you hold about your body and your health. Speak

1. I am sorry- I am sorry that I ignored you (my body) till now.

2. Please forgive me-Please forgive me for eating unhealthy food and not respecting you.

3. Thank you- Thank you that you are with me and have kept me alive till now.

4. I love you –I love you, my body, for everything you have done, is doing and would do to keep me alive and healthy.

This prayer would help you release that guilt and blocked energy from within. Include more of those activities in your daily routine that make you feel strong and uplifted, both physically and mentally. Listen to the stories of good health. Find references to the people who are old and fit enough- those who are enjoying perfect health. Don't listen to the stories of others about various diseases and their aging. I refused to listen to the diseases and ailments of others when I learned this secret to good health.

Listening to the diseases and illnesses of others, you give your mind references. For example, if you have ever heard that by the age you reach 40 or so, your eyesight would not work properly, might not be that clear, you couldn't see clearly, you would not be that active or you would get some disease or ailment. As the subconscious mind is always active and recording such references, these are stored in our mind and as a result, when you cross the age of 40, you will start getting such negative thoughts and emotions that were seeded without any such intention. Always be conscious of what you hear and feed your mind with.

Listen to affirmations of health. There are unlimited videos on YouTube. You could play these affirmations at night on your phone and let them sink into your subconscious mind while you sleep and then, after a few days or months, you would start experiencing the same for yourself too. You could adopt other techniques, as already shared, like charging the water you drink and preparing vision boards.

SCRIPTING YOUR GOOD HEALTH.

Write a script for your good health. Write down how good you feel if you could compete with the young ones. How good do you feel about your fit body? How good do you feel when you exercise? Write down how good you feel when you eat healthy and have no illness or disease in your body. Write down what your emotions would be. Focus all your energy on perfect health.

Focus on the people around you who enjoy perfect health. Make a list of people who inspire you to keep yourself fit. Find out what they do and try to inculcate their fitness habits and diets into your fitness goals. Doing it, you would focus all your energy and attention on a perfect, fit and healthy body and the rule says that where energy flows, it grows. In this way, you are sowing the seed of your perfect, fit and healthy body in your subconscious mind.

Affirm, "The gift of health is keeping me alive."

AFFIRMATIONS FOR HEALTH.

Below is a list of a few health affirmations that could help you.

1. I am fit and fine.
2. I am in perfect shape.
3. I am at my perfect weight.
4. I am energetic.
5. I am always active.
6. I am healthy.
7. I am getting better each day.
8. I am getting fit and losing weight effortlessly.
9. I feed my body only healthy food and drinks.
10. I choose thoughts that create health within me.
11. I am a friend to my body.
12. I am worthy of good health.
13. I listen to what my body says.

14. I only entertain thoughts of good health and wellness.

15. My body is strong and powerful.

16. I have a strong immune system.

17. I have everything I need to live in perfect health.

18. My body knows how to get into its best shape easily and effortlessly.

19. I have everything I need to live in a perfect body.

20. I have a glass skin.

21. I love my personality.

22. I am attractive.

23. I look stunning.

24. I am grateful for my fit and active body.

25. Every cell in my body is healthy.

26. My body heals very quickly.

27. I deserve good health.

28. Health and wellness are mine now.

29. My body and mind are strong.

30. I take care of my mental and physical health.

31. I focus my thoughts on being healthy.

32. I choose to be healthy and happy.

33. I love myself.

34. I love each cell of my body for keeping me alive.

35. I am in perfect health and well-being.

36. I give myself permission to be healthy.

37. I am perfect.

38. I enjoy being healthy, fit and fine.

39. I listen to my body's messages with love.

40. I am filled with love and life.

Happier thoughts lead to a happier, healthier body. Our body has everything in itself to heal. We just need to remove psychological stress, fear and blockages from our body and mind.

I always say that incurable means " curable from within."

Dr. John Demartini
from the book "The Secret".
By Rohnda Byrne.

Richness of Relationships

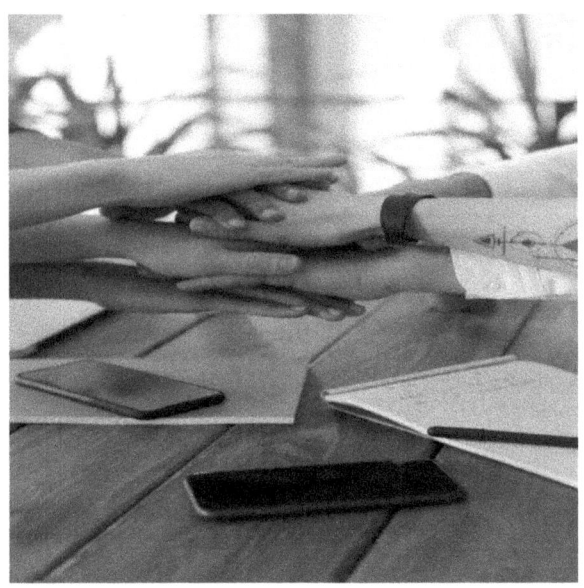

"Everyone is mean, "I cannot trust anyone," "People always hurt me," "No one loves me," "No one understands me" and "No one likes me." Are these your beliefs about yourself and others? Then be prepared to experience them in your life. Your external world is just a projection of your internal world.

If you believe others to be mean, untrustworthy or hurtful to you, you are going to end up attracting such people into your life. Your external world is just mirroring back to your internal world, what you believe about yourself and others. You will always attract to you what you believe is true for yourself. Work on changing your inner dialogue about others. Change the story of your relationship with others in your mind. Think more about loving, trustworthy and supportive people around you. I always affirm, "I am surrounded by loving, kind and supportive people. "I repeat this affirmation a number of times each day and it has worked miraculously in my life. When you affirm such positive statements repeatedly, you become the attraction point for such loving, supportive and kind people around you and those who are not aligned with these words will automatically not be in your life anymore.

Never think wrong about anyone because telepathy works. Your negative thoughts are an energy that reaches the other person and as a result, the other person too starts feeling the same emotions as you. So, if you have negative emotions for someone, instead of thinking and feeling negatively about the other person and focusing your energy on what wrong they said or did to you, just release your energy by focusing on their positive personality traits and the lessons you learned by being around that person. Never gossip about others, as it's low vibrational energy and in return, it will bring back to you only the low vibrational incidents. Instead, focus all your energy on "How could I help others?" Asking this would shift your energy toward yourself. Think of doing some acts of generosity for others for love, peace, happiness and contentment in your life. Never talk badly about anyone. Everyone has their own journey. You never know what the other person is going through. So, just bless the other person and move on. Check yourself often. What is my energy?

What am I talking about? Am I talking badly about others? How would this impact my life? "As you focus, you attract." If you focus on the bad qualities or negatives of another person, you will attract the same for yourself. Asking these questions will give you a clear picture of what exactly you are focusing on and what you will attract in your life.

HO'OPONOPONOPRAYER FOR RELATIONSHIPS.

This prayer for a relationship helps to clear out the blocked energy between you and the other person. Whenever you feel that your relationship with someone is not going well and you want to make it better and forgive that person, start practicing this prayer for a few days to experience its magic. It will free you from all the blocked energy, emotional pain and guilt. By repeating these four sentences, you would be able to clear out that negative energy in your relationship.

1. I am sorry- I am sorry if I ever hurt you with my words or actions.
2. Please forgive me-Please forgive me for that.
3. Thank you-Thank you for being in my life and making me learn new life lessons.
4. I love you- I love you now for who you are.

You can do this prayer for yourself too. When we have negative self-talk with ourselves or when we accept those negative words and phrases from the people around us and block our own energy from flowing, stand in front of the mirror and repeat this prayer 11 to 21 times every day. This prayer would release that blocked energy and you would feel more connected and in love with yourself.

WRITE A GRATITUDE LETTER TO THAT PERSON.

As gratitude is the highest vibration, whenever you feel strong negative emotions like grudges or resentment for someone, try to pen down the good qualities of that person and pay gratitude for being in your life and for all he or she has done for you till date. This will put you in gratitude frequency, which is the high vibrational frequency. You would then be able to feel that love and positivity for that person, which would ultimately result in forgiving and building better relations. The various other techniques, such as vision boards, gratitude messages and charging the water, could also help you manifest better relationships.

BLESS OTHERS.

Give blessings to others. Start blessing everyone around you, including your spouse or partner, colleagues, house help, children and everyone else. Be clear about how you can contribute to your relationships. Do not resist the negative behavior of others, as what you resist will persist. Don't focus on any differences, negative incidents or arguments in your relationship. Always focus on the best moments you share together.

WE ATTRACT WHAT WE ARE, NOT WHAT WE WANT.

Always treat yourself the way you want others to treat you. By treating yourself with love, admiration and appreciation, you emit a strong signal to the universe that you are loved, admired and appreciated. As a result, you attract all the relationships in your life that would make you experience that love, admiration and appreciation. If you want love from others, fill yourself up with love. To attract love from others in your life, do everything that makes you feel satisfied, happy and loved. You attract to your life what you are and not what you want. If you are filled with love, peace and happiness, you will become a magnet to attract the same people and relationships in your life. Fill your cup first, only then will you be able to build strong, loving and long-term relationships with others. If you are not happy with yourself, you can never radiate that happiness on the outside.

PRACTICE SELF LOVE.

Start practicing self-love. Love yourself a bit more each day. Never use any negative words or statements about yourself. Be your own best friend. You can only love and appreciate others if you first love and appreciate yourself. Celebrate being "YOU" each day. Admire and appreciate yourself for who you are and how far you have come. Appreciate yourself for all the hard work you have done-your achievements, struggles, lessons and experiences. Love who you are. Never pass the mirror without giving yourself a compliment or high five, as such little actions of yours would give your subconscious mind a message that you are important, appreciated, admired and loved. When you love yourself, you are then able to give love to others in your relationship. Love is the only force that could make your relationships worthy.

Make a list of things that make you happy. Do them often. Rather, try to do any of them every day. When you feel bad about yourself, you become a magnet to attract more of such bad circumstances, situations and relationships in your life. So, always focus more on your positive aspects. Focus on the good side of yours and when you focus on the good side, you will be able to give love and happiness to your relationships.

"Treasure your relationships, not your possessions."

-Anthony J. D' Angelo
(An Author)

Richness of Money

"If you are born poor, it's not your mistake, but if you die poor, it's your mistake."

-Bill Gates
(An American Philanthropist and Investor)

Are you the one who has heard during your growing years that "Money does not grow on trees" or "Money is the cause of all evil" or "Money is bad" or "Money cannot buy everything" or "Rich people are bad?"

We have all heard such statements about money at some point in our lives. Gradually, during my personal development journey, I learned how these statements affect our relationship with money. I learned that there is abundance in this universe. I learned that money is not the cause of all evil; rather, a lack of money is the cause of all evil. I learned that when we grew up hearing all such negative statements about money, we blocked the flow of money and abundance in our lives. Yes, money cannot buy everything, but money can buy everything on this planet that could be bought with money. Money can buy things that can make you happy. Money is good. We could enjoy a great life if we had an abundance of money in our bank accounts. Money allows us to help others. If we have more than enough for ourselves, we will be able to help others in so many different ways.

As we have already learned, money is energy. Let's say it's listening to such negative statements that money is bad or money is the cause of all evil. Do you feel you will attract it into your life? What would you do if you heard someone talking badly about you? You would definitely start keeping yourself away from that person until you forgive them. The same is the case with money too. The more negative and limiting beliefs you hold about money, the more you have to struggle to earn money. You must have seen many people who are less educated and less intelligent, but they are earning much more than those who are more educated and more intelligent. It is just because their beliefs regarding money are positive and strong enough. We are all programmed since childhood to have all the wrong beliefs about money and in adulthood, we end up struggling to make money for ourselves.

If you have limiting beliefs like "I can't be rich," "I have to work really hard to earn money," or "There is not enough money," then this is what you are going to experience in your life. Start working on your limiting beliefs. Never consider money an evil; otherwise, it will be lost, as you cannot attract what you criticize; rather, always speak good about money.

FALL IN LOVE WITH MONEY.

Money, like everything else, is just an energy. It's all about what beliefs, thoughts and energy you give to the money that will ultimately show up in your life. Every wealthy and rich person has strong and positive beliefs about money. If asked about money, they would say, "Money is good," "Money is freedom, "I love money."

You cannot attract into your life anything that you reject or speak poorly about. You cannot get your child admitted to a top school without money. You need money for that. Right? You need money for the upbringing of your child. You need money for your family. Love, peace and happiness enjoy their own place in our lives, but we cannot have a great life without money. Start becoming conscious of your thoughts and emotions about money. Observe how you think and feel about money on a daily basis. Then start changing your vibrations and your energy toward money. Start falling in love with money. Repeat "I love money and money loves me" every time you hold it in your hands, be it rupees 2, 20, or 2000, as the energy is the same, no matter what the denomination of your money is. Let the money know that you love it. Speak out, "I love you." Say, "Thank you" to money for being in your life.

Find out the various ways to show love to your money. Dance to the tune of the song "Money is coming to me" for 30 consecutive days and feel the change in your energy. You would definitely feel the experience of an increasing flow of money in your life. It's all about the energy we are giving that's coming back to us. Remember, "Like attracts like." Start thinking about the thoughts of abundance and prosperity in your life. When you focus on a lack of money, you will manifest a lack of it only. Focus on being abundant and prosperous. Always feel good about money, even when you are paying your bills. Don't feel the lack of money. Don't feel that you are left with less money. Always pay your bills with gratitude, as you have used those services.

WASH OUT THE WORD, "SPEND MONEY."

Don't fear spending money. Wash out the word "spend money" from your vocabulary. The word "spend" means it's gone. It won't be there anymore. The more you say I am spending money, the more you are dismissing it. Never say I have "spent" money; instead, use the words "circulate" or "invest." To circulate means to come back to the point of origin. It means the money you paid for your electricity bill or for the education of your child will come back and bring more money to you. Repeat, "All the money that I pay returns to me multiplied," or you can use the word "invest" as "invest" means you would get returns on the money you are paying. This means that the money you paid would come back and bring more money along with it.

BLESS YOUR MONEY.

Start blessing your money. Whenever you spend money, affirm that "the money I am paying will come back 10 times." Pay money with the intention of getting back many folds. As money is energy, keeping your money in a bank account and not using it will block the flow of energy. To get money, start giving money. Start circulating it. You can make donations for the needy every month. You can start with a meager amount of Rs 11 or 21 and you could increase the amount gradually.

Bless the money you are earning. Either it is from the business or the job. Be grateful for that business or the job from which you are receiving money in your life, even if it is not your dream job. The more grateful you are, the more you open the doors for abundance and prosperity to flow into your life.

ATTITUDE OF RICH PEOPLE.

Learn the attitude of rich people. Rich people never bargain. They never negotiate with money. When we bargain, we give the impression to our subconscious mind that "I can't afford it." The day I learned, I stopped bargaining. Never ask for the change back. Let the other person keep the change. Rich people don't ask for the change back. Rather, start paying a bit more than the other person asked for. By doing so, you would leave an impression of you being rich and having enough money in the minds of other people and if you could do it with 5 to 10 people each day and transmit the energy of you being a rich person or having more than enough money, could you imagine what would happen? The impression in their minds of you being rich and having enough money would turn out to be your reality. Firstly, you gave that impression to your own subconscious mind by paying a bit more, by not taking the change back, or by not bargaining and with the energy of those 5 to 10 people who felt that you had more than enough money, you would be able to co-create everything for yourself, as the law of the universe says, "Everything is co-created and nothing is a co-incidence."

Never ask for discounts or free gifts. When you ask for discounts or free gifts or expect them, you are giving a command to your subconscious mind that you have limited money or don't have enough. By giving this command, you would attract more of such circumstances into your life, which would prove to you that you don't have enough or have limited money.

To increase the flow of money, keep increasing your value. Do something that would add value to the lives of others and money will follow. Be generous. Think about how you could serve others and pay back to society, as rich people always try to serve and add value to the lives of others.

BE OPEN TO RECEIVE MONEY.

We knowingly or unknowingly reject money. In our Indian culture, many times, when guests come to our home and are willing to pay some amount of money as a token of love, our parents usually refrain or stop the child from taking that money and that's how we learn in our daily lives to say "no" to money that comes our way. The universe works through people. Never reject any money received as a token of love. You attracted it into your life with your own vibrations and frequencies. Whenever any guests give you money, never say "no" to it. Be open to receiving it. Always be in a receiving mode. Don't reject the frequency of money. Receive it with "thanks."

WISH FOR OTHERS WHAT YOU WISH FOR YOURSELF.

Many times, we challenge others for their success or speak poorly about the money or luxuries they enjoy. We usually think that the other person must be adapting some wrong means to achieve success or to buy those luxuries. Never use negative words or statements about others, be it about money, success or luxuries. When you use such negative words and statements for others, you are, in a way, rejecting them for yourself. Instead, be happy for others success; be happy for them buying luxurious cars; and be grateful that you are witnessing such great things happening around you, as this gives evidence to your mind that if they can own it, you too can. The only reason they enjoy that is because they have succeeded in matching the vibration and frequency of that thing to manifest in their lives. Be happy for the success, promotion and good fortune of others to attract the same in your life. The universe works by law.

HAVE YOU EVER BEEN FOR SHOPPING?

Have you ever been shopping? Of course, "yes." You must have been. Have you ever left things, clothes, or other items, saying they were expensive or very expensive? Of course, you must have. Never do that. By saying so, you are giving the subconscious mind the impression that you don't have enough money and can't afford them. Rather than leaving such items and saying that they are expensive, hold them in your hands, feel the feelings of touching them, smell them and imagine yourself enjoying them and then just say "thank you" for this wonderful feeling and put them back on the rack. In this way, you played with the energy of that thing and ordered the universe to deliver it to you and if you succeeded in matching the frequency of that thing, it could be delivered to you. You could receive the same as a gift from someone.

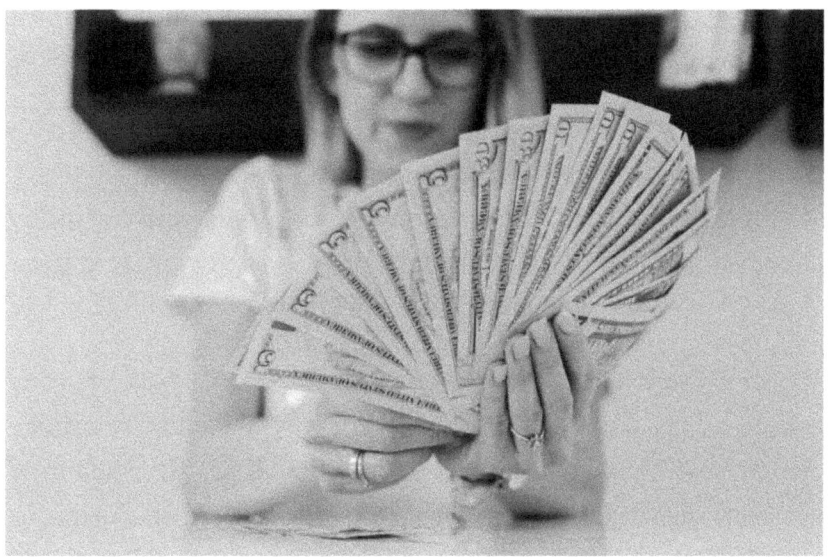

HO'OPONOPONO PRAYER FOR MONEY.

To increase your energy for money, you can practice the Ho'oponopono Prayer. It's a Hawaiian prayer. It's truly a magical prayer. By holding money in your hand, speak out these 4 sentences:

1. I am sorry.
2. Please forgive me.
3. Thank you.
4. I love you.

These four sentences would clear out the blocked energy between you and the money.

"I am sorry" that I didn't respect and love you. I am sorry to think and speak all those negative words and phrases about you (money).

"Please forgive me" for all those wrong words and statements I used for years about you. Forgive me for those limiting beliefs I had about you (money).

"Thank you" for being in my life and for everything I bought and enjoyed because you were with me. Thank you for those unlimited things that I bought and the money that I have used since the day I was born on this planet.

"I Love You" Now that I have realized that it was you who stood by me and helped me in every way, I want to say that I would love to have more of you (money) in my life. I just love you money.

This prayer would help in cleaning out all that blocked energy between you and the money and then proceed to write a "Love letter to money". Writing a "Love letter to money" would make you feel grateful for all the money that you have ever enjoyed in your life. It would increase your vibrations for money and you would be able to attract more of it into your life. The purpose of writing the "Love letter to money" is to match the frequency of money and invite more money into your life.

VISUALIZATION TECHNIQUE.

Start visualizing yourself living in abundance and prosperity. Feel the emotions and feelings of your new version, which has an abundance of money in the bank account. Imagine how beautiful your life would be. Imagine yourself buying luxury items. Imagine yourself helping others with your money. Imagine yourself driving your dream car. Imagine yourself living in your dream home. Feel the emotions of your rich and abundant "you."

AFFIRMATIONS FOR MONEY.

To manifest more money in your life, start practicing money affirmations. To reprogram your subconscious mind for abundance and prosperity, listen to money affirmation songs. You could easily find them on YouTube. Dance to your favorite money song. Let the universe know how abundant and prosperous you are with your feelings. You could also play the affirmations while sleeping because when we are sleeping, our conscious mind is also sleeping and cannot interfere and these affirmations would go straight into the subconscious mind. You can also use various other techniques for money manifestations, as already discussed.

Below is a list of a few affirmations that would help you change your limiting beliefs: Choose any five affirmations that appeal to you, repeat them every day and experience an increased flow of money in your life.

1. I welcome money into my life.

2. I am a magnet for abundance and prosperity.
3. Money flows to me easily and effortlessly.
4. I get paid to exist.
5. Money is constantly finding me everywhere.
6. I am the wealthiest and healthiest version of myself.
7. I am now enjoying financial freedom.
8. I am now enjoying multiple sources of income.
9. I now have more than enough money in my bank account.
10. I live a life of abundance.
11. I am in harmony with the universe.
12. I am a magnet for success.
13. My bank account grows every day.
14. Money finds me wherever I go.
15. I am on the path to financial freedom.
16. I am rich.
17. I am a money magnet.
18. I am a multimillionaire.
19. I am abundant.
20. I am a successful person.
21. I am living a luxurious life.

22. Money comes to me through expected and unexpected sources.

23. My income is always increasing.

24. I am open and receptive to all the wealth in my life.

25. I am enjoying multiple sources of income now.

26. I am independent and self-sufficient.

27. I attract opportunities that create more wealth.

28. I have a growing financial flow.

29. I experience wealth as a key part of my life.

30. I am always discovering new sources of income.

31. I am known as a prosperous individual.

32. I now have the attitude of a successful and rich person.

33. I am intelligent and focused.

34. I am a rich person.

35. Money loves my company.

36. Wealth is my birthright.

37. I invest and manage my money wisely.

38. I have an abundance mentality.

39. I allow money to freely enter my life.

40. I am worthy of a wealthy life.

I couldn't forget to mention here the famous money affirmation by Bob Proctor that is repeated by some of the most successful people, which is "I am so happy and grateful now that money comes to me in increasing quantities through multiple sources on a continuous basis."

Be open to abundance and prosperity. There is nothing lacking in this universe. The only lack that exists is in our own thoughts. So, work on your limiting beliefs and let this universe unfold its magical ways to make you experience your dream life.

> *"Money is the sixth sense that makes it possible to enjoy the other five."*
>
> *-W.Somerset Maugham*
> *(An English Writer)*

Richness of Career:

As we know, our thoughts create our reality, so instead of criticizing, crying and complaining about the job or business that you are in and are not happy with, be grateful that it is helping you to make a living. Be conscious of feeling good about your job or business each day to experience the progress you want in your career. Check your beliefs about your career.

Do you believe that you don't deserve that higher post that one of your colleagues enjoys because you are not that well educated, or do you believe that you are stuck in your job and finding a better job is not possible for you? Do you feel your boss would never promote you? Or do you feel you are not worthy of a salary hike? Do you fear promotion because with it comes more responsibility? Release such negative beliefs. Work on your beliefs, as that is exactly what is going to manifest as your experience in life. Instead, reprogram yourself with positive thoughts like, "I love myself to grow and learn."

Be clear on what you want. Work on your limited beliefs regarding your job, business and career. Check your communication with yourself. Always focus on your success rather than your failures. Don't affirm the negative beliefs of others, like "There is too much competition," "Everyone is better than you," or "You can't crack this exam or interview."

Don't let others negative thoughts influence your way of thinking. Always be positive and receptive. Affirm, "I only deserve the best in my career." Never blame anyone for any experience of your life, as what you are manifesting is just mirroring your internal world. The same is the case in your career too. If you see yourself as incapable, incompetent, irresponsible or unintelligent, you will experience the same from your boss, colleagues and others in your professional life.

Work on building empowering beliefs about your career and success. See yourself as capable, competent and responsible enough to handle your professional responsibilities. Practice affirmations to boost your confidence and build positive beliefs about your career. Be kind, supportive and grateful towards everyone in your professional setup. It would, in turn, make your professional relationships stronger and more trustworthy. Focus on building positive and supportive relationships with everyone as opportunities come through people around you.

VISUALIZATION.

Sit down in silence for 15-20 minutes and imagine yourself doing what you love the most. Imagine finding your purpose, following your passion and attracting success, abundance and prosperity in your life.

You could also use a vision board to manifest your dream career.

If you feel that you are not worthy of a good job or business, ask yourself, "Why do I think this way?" "What is that I fear?" "What are my limiting beliefs about my work?" Whatever your position, it's your thinking that got you there. No one is to blame. Work on checking your thoughts and beliefs.

Never criticize the job you are doing. I too used to criticize my job a lot until I realized it was exactly where I needed to be to reach where I want to be. And now I am truly grateful for my job. Be grateful for where you are and work on improving yourself to be where you want to be in your career with a positive mindset.

GRATITUDE LETTER.

Write a thank-you letter for the company, the job, or the business you are in. Thank your job in helping you make money and a living. Thank your job for everything you are enjoying with the money you get from it, be it paying for your child's education, buying groceries, paying rent, electricity bills, shopping and much more. Thank your current job for everything that is possible because of the money you get from that job or business, even though it is not your dream job. Let the universe know how grateful you are for everything that is coming your way through that job and attract into your life more opportunities to succeed in your career with your positive vibrations.

Below is a list of a few career affirmations to help you.

1. I am creating my dream career.

2. Better career opportunities are coming into my life.

3. I have unlimited career opportunities.

4. I owned my position.

5. I am attracting the best and most suitable job for me right now.

6. I am the best at everything I do.

7. I learn new things easily and effortlessly.

8. I am doing what I love.

9. I am a learner.

10. I am dedicated.

11. I am growing in my life in every aspect.

12. I am successful.

13. I am earning money doing what I love.

14. I am living my passion.

15. I am earning a name and fame.

16. I am attracting money by doing what I love the most.

17. I am living my dreams.

18. I enjoyed the best relationship with all my colleagues.

19. I am surrounded by supportive people.

20. I am open to learning something new each day.

21. I am open to opportunities.

22. I am a receiver.

23. I am energetic.

24. I am the best at what I do.

25. I am a person with assets.

26. I am reliable.

27. I am an inspiration.

28. I am a genius.

29. I am relaxed at work.

30. I love my job.

When you repeat such positive statements again and again, you gradually open up new doors for opportunities to flow into your life.

www.ingramcontent.com/pod-product-compliance
Lightning Source LLC
LaVergne TN
LVHW061552070526
838199LV00077B/7010